THE BEGG APPLIANCE AND TECHNIQUE

THE BEGG APPLIANCE AND TECHNIQUE

by **G. G. T. Fletcher** LDS, D.Orth. RCS

Senior Lecturer, Eastman Dental Hospital, 1959–80

WRIGHT·PSG

Bristol London Boston
1981

© G. G. Fletcher,
1 Wimblehurst Road, Horsham,
West Sussex, 1981

Published by John Wright & Sons Ltd, 42–44 Triangle West, Bristol BS8 1EX, England.

John Wright PSG Inc., 545 Great Road, Littleton, Massachusetts, 01460, U.S.A.

British Library Cataloguing in Publication Data
Fletcher, G.G.T.
    The Begg appliance and technique.
    1. Orthodontic appliances
    I. Title
    617.6'43'0028   RK528.B

ISBN 0 7236 0570 X

Library of Congress Catalog Card Number: 81–52684

Printed in Great Britain by
John Wright & Sons (Printing) Ltd,
at the Stonebridge Press, Bristol BS4 5NU

I myself feel that one should not be tied to a dogma if it is a piece of mechanism. If it is a principle that is different.

Mr Harold Macmillan

Preface

This book combines description and review of a well known appliance system. As such it contains some retrospective judgement, but little comment and even fewer ideas that can be claimed as genuinely original.

The opinions expressed have resulted from the sifting and clinical testing of suggestions and recommendations put forward by others in papers, articles, books and through personal communication. It is almost impossible to recognize adequately the contribution made by so many individuals to one's personal knowledge of the subject.

The first debt of gratitude must therefore go to those many who, wittingly, willingly or otherwise, have influenced the contents of this book.

After paying tribute to the many, there remain the few to whom particular thanks are due, notably Dr P. R. Begg himself, without whose inventive capacity the title of this book would be meaningless. His was the original thought and action which generated a new form of appliance and an associated technique. Like other originators, he came to stand in a lonely and exposed position, where he could hope to receive the admiration of the majority whilst, at the same time, expect some criticism from those who are wise after the event.

The validity of any such criticism depends upon whether it is itself wise. If so, a step forward will have been taken; if not, the criticism will be criticised into extinction.

The element of criticism contained in this book is intended to be constructive and certainly not to denigrate the work of Dr Begg, for which many throughout the world are grateful, not only for it's originality but for the stimulus that it has given to orthodontic thought in general.

Finally, I thank those who have assisted in various ways in the compilation of this book. I am indebted to the staff of the Eastman Dental Hospital, London, both past and present, for their encouragement and helpful advice, and to Mr Morgan, of the same hospital, for his photographic assistance.

Last, but not least, I thank Mrs Clare (Vicky) Howarth for painstakingly typing the text.

G.G.T.F.

Contents

Introduction

Many years of painstaking effort have been devoted by Dr P. R. Begg to the development of an appliance and an associated technical application which are alike both viable and practical. This book has been developed from notes originally written to support short courses on the Begg appliance and technique, given by the Eastman Dental Hospital, London.

Area of Applicability of the Begg Appliance and Technique

The Begg appliance is a comparatively new addition to the orthodontic mechanical field. As would be expected with such a relatively new device, a number of technical improvements have already been made to the original components and their assembly. The modifications have been small but significant and have led to greater reliability.

When the Begg appliance and technique were first introduced, initial propaganda to popularize the approach was often based on emphasizing apparent advantages and simplicities in comparison with the edgewise system, whilst at the same time avoiding mention of any disadvantages.

The Begg appliance was customarily described in the context of the treatment of Class II division 1 occlusions, in association with extraction of the first bicuspids. When used in this way, treatment took a form which divided conveniently into three distinct stages, providing thereby an ease of description of deceptive simplicity. These three treatment stages collectively formed the basis of the Begg technique.

In time, there were many who came to an almost instinctive belief that the Begg appliance was only suited to the treatment of Class II extraction cases and that the procedures of Stages 1, 2 and 3 were always deployed in exactly the same manner, regardless of the form of the occlusion.

It is still of initial convenience to describe the use of the appliance in three stages as they apply to the treatment of Class II division 1 occlusions and this book adheres closely to that concept. A time comes, however, when some technical modifications have to be introduced in order to deal with other forms of malocclusion, which include some non-extraction situations and local anomalies.

'Techniques', which must include that of Dr Begg, are susceptible to being employed as magic formulae by the less well informed in order to avoid the inconvenience of having to think. They often provide the answers to routine problems, being based on averages, but for this very reason seldom cover the advent of the unusual. Unusual occurrences are both varied and frequent, due to the nature and extent of human variation itself. Small improvizations may be required which demand thought based on a thorough understanding of basic mechanical principles. (This observation is included to discourage blind adherence to a set of rules, not to encourage wild modification or invention for the fun of the thing.)

The Begg appliance is, like others, a mechanical means to an end. Appliance systems differ in the type of mechanical advantage over tooth movement that they offer to the operator. The Begg appliance differs fundamentally from the edgewise appliance at the most significant point of control, namely the linkage between archwire and bracket. The edgewise appliance employs a rectangular archwire fitted to a rectangular bracket slot which lies in the same plane as the archwire. The Begg appliance employs a round archwire fitted to a bracket slot which is placed at right angles to the plane of the archwire.

The form of control given by the edgewise archwire/bracket combination, is such as to prevent tilting and therefore to promote bodily movement of the teeth. The prevention of the usual tendency for the teeth to tilt produces frictional resistance between archwire and bracket variable in both degree and location.

This often implies, amongst other things, good anchorage; but not necessarily in those regions where resistance to movement is required. Under these conditions, bodily movement versus bodily movement becomes the basis of the anchorage balance. This fact, together with the frictional resistance, may have to be overcome by introducing high force values which can quickly expend the best intra-oral anchorage, with the result that the use of headgear becomes a frequent necessity.

In the Begg appliance the linkage between archwire and bracket is so designed that tilting is permitted, friction and bracket binding are almost eliminated and, in consequence, the forces employed to promote tooth movement need be comparatively light. Indeed, they must be, because control given to the teeth, including those of the anchorage, is more tenuous than that provided by the edgewise appliance and can easily be overtaxed by well intentioned enthusiasm to move teeth more rapidly by the use of forces, acceptable with the edgewise appliance, but excessive for the Begg. The orthodontist's aim, using the Begg appliance, should be steady continuous progress avoiding error. Attempts to go faster through increases in archwire or elastic pressure result in excessive tilting, rolling and general anchorage loss. If forces are kept light, a great stride will have been taken towards avoiding these errors, which might well be difficult to correct, and strain on anchorage will become reduced to a point where extra-oral support is rarely needed.

The frictional problems associated with the edgewise appliance, arise from the comprehensive three dimensional control it provides to the individual tooth. This control allows the use of a wide range of comparatively heavy pressures without penalty. The same control provides the means of recovering from at least some errors of inadvertent and disadvantageous tooth movement, should they happen.

The Begg bracket/archwire relationship reduces not only the frictional problem but also the means to recover from error, should that occur, and allows only the narrowest range of light pressure to be used without the risk of creating those errors.

The edgewise and Begg appliances, therefore, because of the differences in bracket/archwire relationship and form, offer almost opposite approaches to the mechanical movement of teeth. Each can boast advantages not contained in the other. Likewise there are disadvantages to each not represented in the other.

Although there are basic disciplines common to the practice of all banded appliances, it would be wrong to think that the technical procedures, force values or anchorage responses associated with the efficient practice of the edgewise appliance are directly transferrable, *en bloc*, to the Begg appliance. The differences must be learnt and then lived with until practice makes perfect.

Technical Simplicity

The bends and archwire designs used with the Begg appliance are seemingly simple, but no one should be deceived into thinking that managing to achieve these simple archwire shapes is enough. It is not so much the shape of each bend that is important, but the force and the balance of forces that these bends supply. The Begg appliance demands the utmost precision in all its application. Beware the fact that the light round archwire, when wrongly shaped and adjusted, can nevertheless often be applied to the bracket slots without difficulty but inevitably with disastrous consequences.

If the wrong shape and activity are imparted to heavier gauge archwires used with other appliances, the orthodontist may be unable to seat the wire in the bracket channels and thus receive a timely warning of inaccuracy, causing him to rethink and reshape.

The Begg appliance offers comparative technical simplicity and, through its particular archwire/bracket linkage, an ease of tooth movement. The simplicity offered must however be properly supported by thought and sound judgement and not allowed to degenerate into carelessness through inattention to detail; and the ease of tooth movement must not be taken to mean that the only teeth that move easily are those one happens to want to move.

Anchorage

In addition to relative technical simplicity, the Begg appliance offers an economy in the use of intra-oral anchorage. This is brought about, in the first place, through the bodily control given to anchor units, the freedom to tilt offered to the units that are to be moved and the light forces employed. The latter are insufficient to cause rapid movement of the anchorage, yet adequate for continuity of tilting movements.

In the second place, when the time comes to correct the axial inclinations of the tilted units, the forces employed often partially counterbalance one another. When this is not the case, or only partly true, the reciprocal forces from the root movement auxiliaries are born by the dental arch as a unit, not by a section of the dental arch. When inter-maxillary elastics are added, the two dental arches virtually become one unit, the whole being resistant to any displacing force created by the balance of action of the spring auxiliaries.

The total effect leads to the fact that additional anchorage, supplied through headgear, is seldom needed with the Begg appliance. Nevertheless, it would surely be wrong to advise that headgear should never be employed, or that it cannot be used to advantage. Accidents, resulting in anchorage loss, can happen. The provision of additional anchorage should not be routinely obtained by otherwise unjustifiable extraction of further teeth. One would not willingly send sailors to sea with no life-saving apparatus available, on the grounds that ships do not sink often and even when they do, they only sink once.

Versatility

The addition of headgear, on the few occasions when it may be needed, would seem to broaden further another feature of the Begg appliance, namely its versatility.

There are doubtless those who may be critical of a lack, as they see it, of precision placement of the teeth at the conclusion of active treatment with the Begg appliance. They prefer the accuracy and finality of an edgewise result, having enjoyed the power to place teeth to the nearest fraction of a millimetre. They may even have come to believe that a precision instrument automatically endows them and their judgement with matching precision. This is not necessarily the case and the opportunity and freedom offered by the Begg technique for the teeth to settle those last fractions of millimetres naturally, is probably no disadvantage in the long term.

Approach of this Book

In his book, *Begg Orthodontic Theory and Technique* (1977), Dr Begg has described in detail his treatment approach, which is based upon certain hypotheses backed to some extent by his own researches. His work, both practical and theoretical, has proved stimulating to orthodontists, by being, in certain respects, mildly challenging to previous concepts. As a result Dr Begg's ideas have had an influence on fixed appliance techniques in general and outside his own field.

It would be pointless to repeat, in this book, all that Dr Begg has so ably written on his own behalf. Equally, it would amount to gross ingratitude to attempt to destroy the fruits of his labour. Instead, the subjects of the Begg appliance and techniques have been approached in a way which is almost the reverse of the usual. The appliance has been examined for its potential to move teeth conveniently and efficiently. Foremost amongst the ways in which the appliance can be used to this end is the three-stage procedure which has come to be known as 'the Begg technique'. No radical changes have been suggested for the technique, which remains a valid and effective system of treatment for a high percentage of all types of malocclusion. It has, however, been suggested that there are some orthodontic situations in which, if the pure Begg technique is applied, the results, in one respect or another, are likely to fall short of the ideal and where the shortfall could be avoided if the mechanical concepts were to be altered to cover just those few cases.

Some will see these suggestions as interfering with basic simplicity and as challenging the comprehensive suitability of the Begg technique to the treatment of all forms of malocclusion. If, after reading this book, they remain of that opinion, that is their prerogative. No orders are being issued, but some arguments are subscribed to to the belief that, in some circumstances, the standard format of the Begg technique is not enough. The spirit of this observation is not hostile to anyone, nor destructive of the Begg technique itself.

The real bone of contention is not so much that the Begg technique is not enough, but that the theoretical background provided for its support is too much, by being extended beyond logical limits. It is because of this that the potential of the appliance has been examined first and the background theory, although described and discussed, relegated to a secondary consideration.

Theories

The usual approach is to put forward the theory which purports to justify the treatment method and appliance design, with the assertion that all are inseparably linked.

There are three theories:

(1) Dr Begg's concept of normal occlusion, based on his studies of skulls and dentitions of Australian aboriginals (the Theory of Attritional Occlusion);

(2) The Theory of Differential Pressures; and

(3) The employment, in the appliance mechanics, of a modified form of the ribbon arch bracket and light gauge round archwires.

The Theory of Attritional Occlusion

Briefly, Dr Begg has founded his concept of correct occlusion upon his studies of ancient skulls of Australian aboriginals (Stone Age man). He found that their dentitions displayed a considerable amount of attrition, both occlusally and interproximally. The occlusal surfaces of the cheek teeth had been worn away to eliminate cusps and fissures. In the anterior region, the incisors had worn down to their narrower mesio–distal widths whilst, at the same time, moving progressively towards an edge-to-edge relationship. With the elimination of incisor overbite, mesial migration of the mandibular teeth could take place without incurring lower incisor imbrication. The total reduction in arch length resulting from attrition amounted approximately to one bicuspid width either side of both dental arches by the time the aboriginal was twenty years of age. (*Figs.* 1.1 and 1.2).

As the occlusal surfaces wore away, the intermaxillary height was maintained through continued eruption of the teeth.

It is not surprising that, with the elimination of cusps and fissures, it was found that the caries incidence was low by modern standards, nor that, with the mastication of unrefined food, there was little incidence of gingival disease. In addition, with an absence of incisor overbite it was found that the bane of modern post-treatment orthodontics, late lower incisor crowding, was a less frequent occurrence.

In the present day and age, with refined and precooked food having replaced the former rougher diet, there is correspondingly less dental

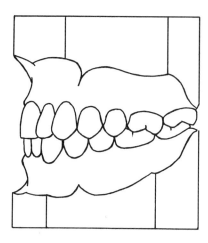

Fig. 1.1. Example of normal occlusion in a young adult of the present day, showing an absence of attrition and possessing upper to lower incisor overlap.

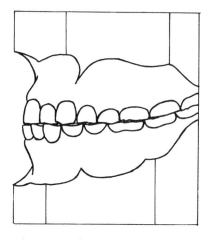

Fig. 1.2. The pattern of a young normal adult occlusion in more primitive times, showing effects of occlusal and interproximal attrition. The dento-alveolar height was maintained by continuous eruption and proximal contact by mesial tooth migration, facilitated by cuspal wear. The incisor relationship became edge-to-edge, thereby reducing the chance of lower incisor imbrication through overbite obstruction.

attrition which, in turn, has lead to increased liability to caries and disorders of the gingivae. Additionally, the absence of attrition in the presence of mesial tooth migration means that dental overcrowding, where it exists, is unrelieved and seen clinically at its worst, particularly in the lower incisor region where the modern overbite prevents their escape into edge-to-edge relationship with the uppers.

These findings accord with those of Miss Corisande Smyth who reported in 1934 her study of Anglo-Saxon skulls found in a burial ground in Bidford-on-Avon. The skulls belonged to the period 500–600 AD. She described the considerable attrition which was displayed in the dentitions of these people, including the prevalence of edge-to-edge incisor relationship. She also found examples of all the well known forms of malocclusion with which we are familiar at the present time. It should not be thought that the ancients were universally equipped with perfect occlusions. An incidental piece of information, attributed to Sir Arthur Keith, arose during the discussion on Miss Smyth's paper; it was observed that, in Bronze Age Britain, edge-to-edge incisor relationship with mild overlap had been common, but the skulls belonging to the time of the Roman occupation had shown marked incisor overlap. In the later Anglo-Saxon period, this overlap was replaced by a return to an edge-to-edge relationship and did not reappear until the reign of Elizabeth I (1558–1603).

Clearly the amount of dental attrition found will vary in accordance with the degree of refinement or otherwise of the regular diet. Tough unrefined food compels the use of strong masticatory forces which will bring about attrition, particularly if grit enters the food, either as sand from a desert environment or particles from millstones.

Dr Begg has used the findings from his study of Australian aboriginal occlusions as a justification for extraction. He argues that if in this present era tooth material is not lost through attrition, it would be reasonable to cause a commensurate reduction artificially. Dr Begg was once a pupil of Dr Angle, who preached a non-extraction approach to orthodontic treatment and was unwilling to recognize possible exceptions. Care must now be taken to ensure that, with the arrival of the opposite approach, the employment of extraction is not also carried beyond logical limits. There will be exceptions to the extraction approach just as there were to the non-extraction concept (*Fig. 1.3*).

Extraction to create space for the accommodation of the remaining teeth of crowded dental arches was written up in the dental literature as long ago as 1802. It was not a new idea even then and certainly is not so now. The issue remains where it was and is self justifying in circumstances

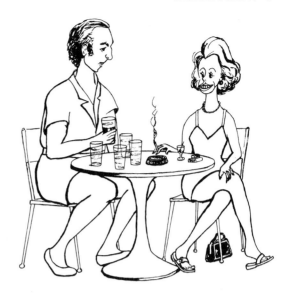

Fig. 1.3. Depicted here are two holiday makers who, when younger, were both orthodontic patients. The one received treatment in a school which believed in the 'always extract' principle, the other in a school tied to the 'never extract' philosophy. From the point of view of facial aesthetics, might it not have been better if each had received the treatment of the other?

which offer no other way of obtaining a stable treatment result of quality.

The anchorage demands made by a particular appliance should not always be met by resort to extraction, even in the interests of uniformity and apparent simplicity, if those demands can be met another way.

Reference should be made to Dr Begg's own views on the implications of Stone Age man's attritional dentition to the employment of extraction as part of orthodontic treatment. The above summary is too brief to do justice to his work and might be thought by some to be biased.

The Theory of Differential Pressures

The theory of Differential Pressures in its original form was described by Dr Begg in an article in the *American Journal of Orthodontics* (1956). His observations were based to a large extent on the work of Storey and Smith and their experiments on tooth movement response to different pressure applications.

Broadly, it had been suggested that there was a range of light pressures which would cause teeth to move at an optimum rate and with minimal disturbance of the supportive tissues. Pressures below this range would produce a slow rate of response, whilst those above incurred a reaction within the bone support, sometimes referred to as 'undermining resorbtion', which also had the practical effect of retarding tooth movement.

When these principles were applied to the Begg technique, the force of the inter-maxillary elastic ligatures used in Stage 1 of treatment, was kept light so that the upper labial segment was retracted whilst the lower anchor molars exhibited almost negligible mesial movement. Later, if it was required that the residual extraction spaces should be closed, largely by mesial movement of the posterior teeth, the elastic ligature force was increased so that the upper anteriors with their relatively small root area received an excess of pressure sufficient to delay their movement, whilst the posteriors moved forward. This meant that the operator had some measure of control over the final antero–posterior positioning of the dental arches.

There is no doubt that this facility to position the dentition through varying the relative resistance to movement of the posterior or anterior segments of the arches, is a valuable asset of the Begg appliance. There is also little doubt that heavy orthodontic forces have a different effect on the supportive bone than light ones. In practical terms, it is the heavy elastic forces which cause undue rolling, rotation and elevation, as well as anchorage loss, when tooth movement finally comes about after initial delay. Heavy inter-maxillary forces can easily overcome the molar anchorage control, which is provided in the case of the Begg appliance by a small gauge round wire in a comparatively large round buccal tube, with only the archwire anchor bend to prevent tilting. This control mechanism cannot be expected to withstand heavy forces reliably.

The increase of the anchorage resistance of either the anterior or posterior teeth, at the discretion of the operator when using the Begg appliance is brought about less by varying the force application, than by varying the distribution of the force.

If the teeth of the upper labial segment are permitted to tilt freely they can be retracted by inter-maxillary elastics which supply a force just sufficient for the purpose, but insufficient to move the anchor molars, which are controlled against tilting or rotating by the archwire anchor bend. In the circumstances, the crowns of the teeth of the upper labial segment move palatally and their root ends labially in a tilting motion, whereas the lower first molars have to move bodily with the pressure confined to one side of their roots. In this way the balance of crown movement favours the upper anterior teeth which will be seen to move considerably, with little reciprocal response from the lower posteriors.

If, using the same inter-maxillary force, the teeth of the upper labial segment are compelled to move bodily, through the application of vertical spurs or root torque auxiliaries, the crowns of these teeth will move less, over a prescribed period, than when tilting was permitted. If, in conjunction with this action, the posterior anchor bends are slightly reduced and the inter-maxillary force is increased, the result becomes one of relatively greater mesial movement of the lower posteriors.

The institution of bodily control at one end of the dental arches, either upper or lower, whilst allowing comparative freedom of movement at the other, enables the appliance operator, when using inter- or intra-maxillary elastic ligatures, to control the antero–posterior positioning of the dentition.

Perhaps it could fairly be said that, because of the importance of the bodily control element over that of force values in controlling the balance of movement, the theory of Differential Pressures should perhaps be altered to one of Differential Distribution of Pressures. The principle involved is not new, but it so happens, with the round archwires associated with ribbon arch brackets which constitute the Begg appliance, greater facility is offered to use the principle to better advantage than that given by many other appliance systems.

Light Gauge Archwires and Ribbon Arch Brackets

The use of light gauge 0·016 in working archwires promotes long continuous action in tooth movement whilst keeping force values down at all times below that which might cause pain or discomfort to the patient. It should, perhaps be added that this insurance is not automatic. It is still possible, even with such a light archwire, to introduce local forces sufficient to promote pain and, subsequently tooth mobility, unless care is taken with adjustment. The long action of the archwire assists avoidance of frequent removal for adjustments. The anchorage control afforded is adequate so long as force applications are kept light.

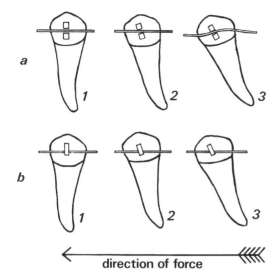

a

1 2 3

b

1 2 3

← direction of force ⟵⟪⟪⟪

Fig. 1.4. The natural response of a tooth to the application of a force to the crown and in the direction of the arrow, is one of tilting. Brackets with slots in the same plane as the archwire (*a*), prevent tilting and consequently cause bracket binding through friction (2) which increases as the archwire flexes (3). Ribbon arch brackets with a vertically placed slot (*b*) permit tilting with the minimum of friction between bracket and archwire.

The ribbon arch bracket, which has a vertically placed archwire slot as opposed to the horizontal slot of an edgewise bracket, forms a free hinge attachment for bucco–lingual tooth movement and also permits freedom for teeth to tilt when moved mesio–distally. When placed in a vertically slotted bracket, the archwire controls the respective heights of the teeth and prevents rotation.

The alliance of the light round archwire and the vertically slotted bracket makes it possible to obtain rapid general alignment using light forces with minimal anchorage expenditure in the early stages of treatment. Unlike the horizontally slotted bracket, the bracket with a vertical slot promotes less friction and locking with the archwire.

Horizontally slotted brackets, such as those employed in edgewise techniques, are inclined to lock with the archwire so that bodily movement is unavoidable (*Fig. 1.4*). The locking can occur at either end of the dental arch, so that inter- and intra-maxillary forces have bodily resistance to overcome at both ends of their action. This implies the use of relatively heavy forces and similar amounts of movement of the anterior and posterior units, which results in the easy expenditure of available intra-oral anchorage. Appliances using horizontally slotted brackets must necessarily obtain the required anchorage largely from extra-oral sources and be associated with an extensive use of headgear. The expectation with the Begg appliance, employing vertically slotted brackets, is for rare use of headgear through more conservative use of intra-oral anchorage.

An example of bracket binding and locking using plain archwires and inter-maxillary elastics is given in *Figs.* 1.5. *a, b* and *c*. The example is not intended to represent actual clinical practice but to give an indication of what could happen if the Begg technique were to employ the wrong type of bracket.

Objectives

It is hoped that a readable, as well as instructive, account of the Begg appliance and technique has been provided and that, through the medium of this book, a basis for sound practice with the Begg appliance and technique will be acquired. New technical modifications and differences in personal approach may be introduced with the passage of time, but the fundamental principles can be expected to remain the same. The main objective of the book is to describe and discuss the appliance as a means to an end, i.e. as a mechanical means of carrying out any reasonable programme of tooth movement which the orthodontist concerned considers suitable for the case under treatment.

Such suitable programmes may well include extraction of units and the subsequent movement of teeth for which the Begg technique is wholly appropriate. The technique has consequently been described in full, but at intervals in this text the suitability of the basic Begg technique and its background theory have been called into question in relation to specific treatment situations. Alternative approaches have been suggested, none without the backing of clinical trial, which could increase the scope of the appliance. The occasional use of headgear with an accompanying redesign of archwires may upset the purists, but the observations have been made for whatever they may ultimately be thought to be worth.

Line diagrams have been preferred to photographs, wherever possible, because the latter often disappoint when examined for extreme detail such as that involved in the composition of a fixed appliance.

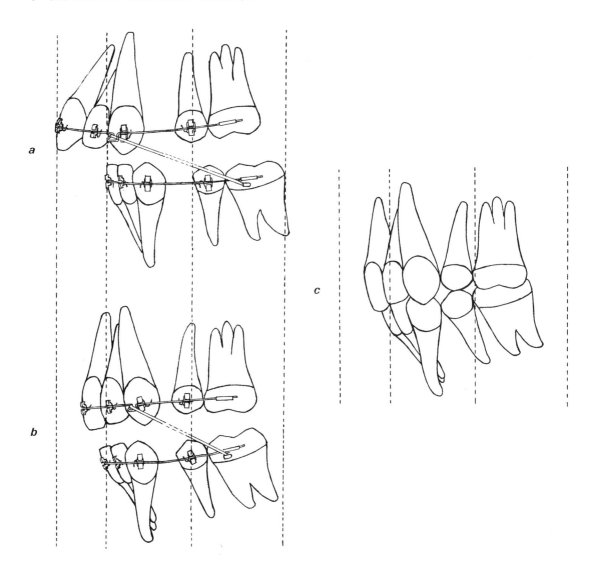

Fig. 1.5*a*, Hypothetical example to demonstrate an effect of bracket binding. If plain archwires, containing no adjustment bends or loops, were to be used in association with an edgewise style of bracket and Class II elastics applied, the upper anteriors would attempt to tilt palatally, whilst the lower posterior teeth try to tilt mesially.

b. As a result of the mechanics shown in *Fig.* 1.5*a*, locking between brackets and archwire would occur amongst the upper anteriors, notably the cuspids, and at the edges of the lower bicuspid brackets and molar tubes. Bodily resistance to the elastic pull is consequently built up anteriorly and posteriorly. The frictional locking amongst the lower posteriors means that the continued application of the intermaxillary elastics would move not only the lower posterior teeth but also the entire lower archwire, causing displacement of the lower incisors labially. The vertical component of elastic force causes an increased forward cant of the occlusal plane, at the same time supplementing any already existing depressive force on the lower incisors. The root ends of these teeth will be moved lingually and their crowns labially.

c, The result of continuation of the process shown in *Fig.* 1.5*b* is an example of a loss of anchorage, in that the entire occlusion has been positioned too far to the labial, with the expectation of instability and relapse. The vertical broken lines help tooth movement interpretation through the three stages shown. In the use of edgewise mechanisms, compensatory mechanics can be added to eliminate the unwanted effects of bracket binding; but these do not remove the fact of bodily versus bodily balance of intra-oral anchorage which results from both archwire and bracket slots being in the same plane. Intraoral anchorage becomes expended early and it will be found that, in a high proportion of treatments employing edgewise mechanisms, additional anchorage will have to be supplied from extra-oral sources.

Case reports have been omitted for a number of reasons, not least that when fully documented each demands much space, and the display of a suitable number would consequently swell the size and cost of this book without adding a commensurate instructional value. There exists plenty of documentary evidence of the effectiveness of the Begg appliance when allied to appropriate skills and to other tooth movement systems described in the following text. Mirror images of these would seem superfluous.

The decision to minimize the contribution of photography to illustration and omit case reports was not taken lightly, any more than was the decision to include some material on the development of Class I and Class II division 2 occlusions. The inclusion of the latter may be judged by some to be irrelevant in a book, ostensibly devoted to the mechanics of an appliance: the object of this inclusion was to reassert the fact that human variation is extensive and that the inter-relation of a number of minor variations can nonetheless have a far reaching effect on the occlusion. The reader will be reminded that the orthodontist does not deal with one or two well worn sets of averages, but can be confronted with unusual situations, so easily forgotten until presented as a clinical fact.

Some criticism will doubtless be made of the juxtaposition within this book of clinical fact, partially substantiated theory and outright conjecture. It is difficult to avoid such a mixture when so much in orthodontics is based on clinical opinion and so little on fact scientifically proven beyond doubt. There can be no argument about the latter, but argument is endless over opinions developed from the clinical experience of individuals: some such opinions are held with a fervour which would do justice to a religious fanatic.

Orthodontics is still in the process of a transition from being a subject largely based on clinical intuition and consequent 'beliefs', to one increasingly supported by scientific fact. Given time, orthodontists will come to prove more of their contentions beyond doubt. In the meantime there will be much that remains hypothetical.

It is hoped that a spirit of tolerance will be shown by the reader towards opinions expressed in this book which may differ from his own. It is probably in no way disadvantageous that this work has been compiled not in the manner of a salesman persuasively purveying the latest faultless product but from the viewpoint of a critical consumer with fifteen years of practical experience with the goods.

There are no faultless orthodontic appliances. Any hint of criticism of the Begg appliance or technique expressed could be levelled in equal measure at any rival method.

The successful use of a given appliance will be based on an understanding of the underlying principles. These can be taught; but the exact practical application of the principles requires a measure of the art of the craftsman, or craft of the artist, which are qualities of the individual and cannot be taught.

Chapter 2

Case selection and preliminary treatment procedures

Case Selection

The Begg appliance offers a comprehensive mechanical system for the handling of tooth movement and therefore cannot be considered as unsuited to the treatment of any form of mal-occlusion.

It is probably true to say that the method will operate at its most effective in association with extractions which provide a margin of excess space. The theory of Stone Age man's attritional dentition gives a plausable excuse to create space by extraction, thus producing the desired situation for the best operation of the mechanics. Nevertheless, the Begg appliance can be used successfully without extractions in suitable circumstances.

Cases to be treated by the Begg appliance will not differ in the main to those selected for treatment by other banded techniques, the principle criteria for which are:

(1) The tooth movements required are such as to demand the forms of control given by banded appliances and cannot be achieved to an adequate standard by simpler methods;

(2) The ultimate stability of the treated occlusion is in doubt, unless root movements accompany the repositioning of the crowns, thereby demanding the mechanics for the purpose;

(3) The patient's interest in his personal appearance and health is such as to have ensured a high standard of oral hygiene which gives promise of future cooperation and the maintainance of regular attendance over the prescribed treatment period;

(4) The above interest can be matched by an actual practical ability, in relation to personal circumstances, to be able to attend regularly at prescribed intervals over the treatment period; and

(5) The parent (in the case of a schoolchild) and patient have been given to understand precisely the nature and duration of the proposed treatment and what is required of each if success is to be achieved.

It would be probably sound advice to those fresh to the use of the Begg appliance and technique, even if experienced with alternative methods, to begin by treating straightforward and relatively simple cases. The more complex situations, where there is little or no margin for mechanical error or anchorage misassessment, should not be tackled until all the fundamentals of the new technique have been thoroughly mastered.

Banding, Bracket Positioning and Auxiliary Band Attachments

The highest standards of accuracy are demanded for the chance of success with all banded techniques, but at no point in treatment is this factor more urgent than during the preliminary banding and bracketing procedures. No amount of time or effort spent in obtaining the best fitting of bands or positioning of brackets will be wasted. Failure to do so results in frequent need to recement or remake bands, unnecessary compensatory archwire adjustments, breakdown in the continuity of treatment through the breakdown of the apparatus itself, associated perhaps with ulceration, decalcification etc. In such ways does overall treatment time become greatly extended beyond that strictly necessary in better ordered circumstances. The bands are there throughout treatment and, if faulty, will adversely affect all stages until the faults have been corrected.

Bands and brackets are fitted with the following intentions:

(1) To obtain optimal fit and positioning on the tooth surface;

(2) To provide a control medium for teeth to be moved;

(3) To provide a control medium for teeth acting as anchorage;

(4) To provide support to the attached archwire in areas where the latter is liable to distortion;

(5) To provide protection for enamel surfaces in areas liable to decalcification;

(6) To minimize the number of visits required for the work to be carried out, consistent with the patient not being overtaxed by undue time in the dental chair on any one occasion;

(7) To avoid as far as possible the use of mass separation which can be painful to the patient the work to be carried out in the order that best suits this aim.

(8) To avoid repetition of the use of separators, bands and attached brackets should be cemented into place on completion whenever possible.

It should be possible, with the above intentions, to fit bands, brackets and the first set of archwires, in two visits of reasonable duration, if the order of procedure is properly thought through. The banding of second bicuspids can be omitted at this stage.

Much well-intentioned advice has been offered as to the order in which the teeth should be banded, based on average conditions. It seems redundant to quote these, since patient circumstances and oral conditions are so variable as to make individual assessment the rule rather than the exception.

In the treatment of Class II division 1 with extraction of first bicuspids, upper and lower left 6 3 2 1 and right 1 2 3 6 are initially banded and archwires placed. As soon as possible thereafter the second bicuspid bands are added.

It is sometimes advised that the banding of second bicuspids is optional in the first stage of treatment of a first bicuspid extraction case. Since this implies a reduction of work load, the rule is usually interpreted that it is never necessary. On the contrary, the otherwise long length of unsupported archwire is reduced by the presence of second bicuspid bands, brackets and bypass clamps. A measure of protection is provided to the archwire and, by assisting the direction of leverage of the anchor bends through support to the archwire against buccal rolling, firmer bodily control over

the anchor molars is obtained. These advantages are of prime importance in the lower arch.

Second lower bicuspid bands should not, however, be placed, if their brackets happen to contact the distal of the buccal cusps of the uppers, whilst in a Class II relationship and when Class II traction is being used. They should be placed as soon as the relationship has been corrected and the obstruction overcome.

Second bicuspids bands should, in all circumstances, be fitted before the final act of space closure, in order to avoid the possibility of overclosure and the possible exclusion of these teeth from the dental arch.

In view of the necessity to employ uprighting springs and spurs to correct axial inclinations in the later phases of treatment with the Begg appliance and in view of the fact that these may closely overlie the enamel surfaces, there are some who deem it advisable to protect the tooth surface against the threat of decalcification, by extending the bands gingivally to cover the areas where the auxiliaries are to be placed.

This action is most pertinent in respect of cuspids and bicuspids and in instances where either the structure of the enamel, or the patient's oral hygiene standard, is in doubt.

Brackets

High flange brackets are preferred to the taper flange, since the former possess a wider welding surface which makes them less liable to distortion. The taper flange bracket could be too readily distorted, leading either to release of the archwire or to frictional binding (*Fig. 2.1j*).

The best of the high flange brackets in current use, have been made of slightly thicker metal than some of their predecessors which reduces the possibility of damage or alterations to the size of the archwire slot through distortion. The same increase in metal content has produced some brackets which are broader at the base of the slot than many of the earlier patterns.

Much has been said in favour of the importance of the one point coupling between archwire and bracket which, it is claimed, assists the easy tilting of the teeth. This is true, but the same factor also permits the easy relapse of teeth following root repositioning in the later phases of treatment, unless the root movement auxiliaries are kept in place. It is desirable to remove these auxiliaries

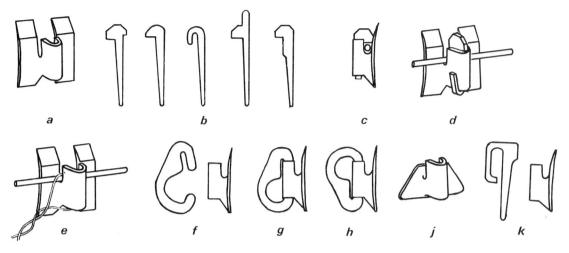

Fig. 2.1. Examples of brackets and bracket to archwire attachment. *a*, The high flange bracket. *b*, Lock pins styles. *c*, Lateral view of bracket and safety lock pin, showing latitude given to an 0·016 in archwire in a 0·020 in slot. *d*, Archwire pinned to bracket. *e*, Method of obtaining firm fixation by wire ligature. One end must emerge through the same channel as the archwire. *f*, The bypass clamp before attachment to the bracket. *g* & *h*, The clamp in position to hold the archwire either high or low in relation to the bracket, in accordance with the dictates of the clinical situation. *j*, The delta wing brackets, now superseded because of the inadequacy of the welding areas. *k*, An alternative to the bypass clamp.

as soon as their purpose has been fully accomplished in order to re-establish better oral hygiene in the areas relatively inaccessible by their presence.

An 0·020 in retaining archwire, which precisely fills the bracket slot, can be used in the final stages of treatment. This archwire will maintain tooth alignment in the horizontal and vertical dimensions and will also ensure against mesio–distal relapse of previous root paralleling, but only if it is ligated or pinned tightly into a bracket slot of adequate mesio–distal breadth.

In the earlier stages of treatment, when free tilting of the teeth is required, the same bracket permits this action so long as a safety lock pin is used.

A variety of Begg brackets and lock pins are made by various manufacturers. It is inadvisable to use the brackets from one source in conjunction with pins from another, since the two components may not coordinate. It should be seen that brackets and pins, not only emanate from the same source but also belong to the same series.

Bracket Positioning

The brackets are placed in the centre of the band viewed mesio–distally, whilst in the vertical dimension, they should be placed within the margins of the band, avoiding having any part, particularly the slot, overhang the edge. The bracket slots should open towards the gingival side of the bands.

Care should be taken that no roughness results from welding the flanges. The surfaces of the flanges must be smooth in order to avoid any possible friction when in contact with the archwire.

The offsetting of brackets towards the mesial or distal in the case of rotated teeth is often advocated, particularly for buccal teeth, the object being to effect over-rotation and to maintain this position once carried out. The amount of offsetting for this purpose should only be slight (*Fig. 2.2*).

In order to avoid eventual extrusion or intrusion of individual teeth, the brackets and bands must be placed at coordinated heights. Unless great care is taken over this matter, the result will be impairment of treatment progress and/or a poor aesthetic and functional outcome, due to uneven incisal edge and occlusal levels (*Fig. 2.3*).

Measurements are taken from the bracket slot to the cusp or incisal edge. Many attempts have been made to advise a universally applicable set of measurements, but once again, individual variation makes these something of an academic exercise.

Brackets and band attachments should not be

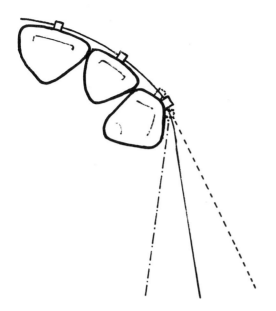

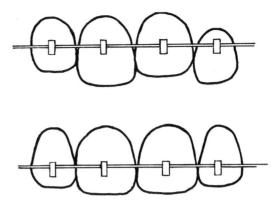

Fig. 2.3. Correct and incorrect bracket heights on the incisor teeth and the effects on the orientation of the incisal edges. Correct relative bracket positioning is no less important for the buccal teeth and for the dental arch as a whole.

Fig. 2.2. Mesio—distal positioning of brackets. The point midway between the mesial and distal margins of the tooth will often be correct, but canines need particular attention. Wrong placement of the brackets of these teeth can result in their inadvertent rotation together with an expansion or contraction of the distal ends of the archwire. The canine eminence is often a little mesial of dead centre of the tooth. If the canine is rotated prior to treatment the distal ends of the archwire will be affected in the same manner, although the bracket may be correctly positioned. Undue and unwanted lateral pressure on the molar should be reduced by archwire adjustment.

placed too near the gingival tissues because stagnation areas and trauma might be provoked once archwires and auxiliaries are fitted. Conversely, damage may result to the attachments or archwires if placed too near the incisal edge or cusp. A compromise must be found to suit the individual patient. This usually amounts in practice to a distance of 3—4 mm from the base of the bracket slot to the incisal edge in the case of the lower anteriors and 4—5 mm for the upper anteriors, including the cuspids.

In the case of the buccal teeth, the measurement is slightly increased over that of the cuspid by not more than a millimetre per unit, as one proceeds posteriorly. This will apply to the position of the buccal tube on the first permanent molar and will result in both it and the second bicuspid bracket being placed well to the gingival.

Measurement in the case of the buccal tube, is taken from mesial opening to the summit of the mesio—buccal cusp of the molar. Antero—posteriorly the tube should be placed so that this opening is directly above or below the mesio-buccal cusp, according to whether it is upper or lower. The tube should lie parallel with the occlusal surface. When these rules are applied, the archwire should emerge so as to lie just to the buccal of the bicuspid teeth, unless the molar is rotated or the bicuspid displaced.

In this matter of bracket height coordination, the upper lateral incisor may become an exception. If this tooth, as is usually the case, is relatively small, it may be in the interests of aesthetics that its incisal edge be not in line with those of the central and cuspid, but slightly elevated above that level. In which case, the distance of the bracket slot to the incisal edge will be less than that of the central by the amount its edge is to be above that of the central.

From the foregoing information, it can be deduced that the buccal attachments are placed progressively away from the occlusal and nearer the gingival, by very small amounts per unit, from the anterior to the posterior of both dental arches (*Fig.* 2.4).

The above arrangement tends to encourage depression of the anterior teeth and elevation of the posteriors. More important, a degree of protection is offered to the vital posterior anchor bends by keeping them, as far as possible, away from occlusal forces and consequent damage.

Although the arrangement implies that the molar tubes are well to the gingival, there is no call

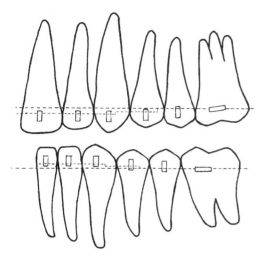

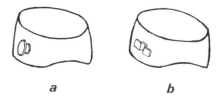

Fig. 2.5. *a*, The lingual button. *b*, The lingual cleat.

Fig. 2.4. The escalation of bracket positions towards the occlusal, working from posterior to anterior. The arrangement assists incisor depression, whilst the relatively gingival placement of the molar tubes keeps the archwire anchor bends away from occlusal forces.

for them to be inserted into the soft tissue, or placed in such close proximity that stagnation and inflammation result. Molar tubes located too far gingivally may also result in the posterior of the archwires intruding into the soft tissue immediately behind the tubes.

The position of the gingival margin in the molar region, relative to the teeth, is variable and should not be used as a measure for the placement of the molar tube. The molar tube should be coordinated in height with the second bicuspid bracket. Absence of coordination will demand, in the later stages of treatment, compensatory height adjustment bends, or vertical offsets, in the main archwire. After the second bicuspid bracket slots have been fully engaged by the archwire, the relatively large lumen of the molar tube, coupled with the continued need for mildly active anchor bends, automatically compels small compensatory archwire offsets in the vertical dimension; but it is detrimental to general appliance stability to allow those bends to become extravagant in size.

Lingual Buttons and Cleats

Many orthodontists routinely add lingual cleats to molar, bicuspid and cuspid bands at the outset of treatment (*Fig. 2.5*).

There will often be adequate clinical crown

available for the purpose but not infrequently, particularly in the case of the lower bicuspids, there is little tooth surface on the lingual aspects on which to place the cleats in such a way that they are neither exposed to damage from occlusal forces nor yet intruded into the gingival tissues. The presence of cleats over long periods can be detrimental to the health of the gingivae.

It would seen advisable to restrict the use of buttons and cleats to those occasions when there is no alternative. Molar crossbites, rotation of cuspids and bicuspids and, in some instances, the need to tie back or tie together to prevent either relapse following retraction and rotation or space reopening following closure, are the principal examples. Any such requirement can and should be forseen at the treatment planning stage.

Not infrequently there is no real need for the use of either lingual buttons or cleats.

When correcting molar crossbite by cross elastic between the lingual of the upper and the buccal of the lower molar, many prefer to place two buttons or cleats on the upper molar, one under the mesial and the other under the distal lingual cusp. The elastic engages both so that the possibility of unintentional rotation is minimized.

If buttons are preferred, they may be prevented (when not in use) from causing irritation to the tongue by the placement of a single Alastic ring on each.

It should be realized that lingual cleats on the upper cuspids can stultify retraction of either the cuspids themselves or the upper labial segment, through contact interference with the tips of the lower cuspids. In these circumstances, not only will tooth movement be interrupted but also the cleats themselves will be damaged, making it desirable to fit them, when needed, at a later stage of treatment.

See also note on Direct Bonding added in proof (page 165).

Chapter 3

Aims and practical procedures for the treatment of Class II first bicuspid extraction cases (Stage 1 treatment)

The basic mechanics of the Begg appliance and the principles of the related technique are perhaps best understood if initially described in the context of the treatment of Class II division 1 occlusions following first bicuspid extraction. The majority of mechanical components are brought into use when treating such malocclusions, which leads to a comprehensive description. The differences and modifications necessary to the treatment of other forms of occlusion thereafter become easier to understand.

The objectives of the first stage of treatment are as follows:

(1) To obtain general alignment, eliminating bucco–lingual displacement and rotation;
(2) To correct vertical discrepancies (levelling);
(3) To reduce overbite to edge-to-edge incisor relationship, inclusive of—
(4) Reduction of overjet; and
(5) To correct the relationship of the buccal occlusion to Class I.

Preliminary Aims in Stage 1 Treatment

Items (1) and (2) above are primary objectives with all banded appliances. Before embarking on the remainder, thought should be given in the case of the Begg apparatus to the possible adverse effects of friction which may result from the procedures of general alignment. In treatments involving correction of severe rotations, or other forms of marked tooth malposition, considerable friction may develop between archwire and bracket. In some such instances, it might be politic to eradicate the worst of the malalignment before attempting to reduce overbite and overjet with Class II elastics. Judgement depends on where the friction develops and on whether or not it causes notable interference to either the free sliding of the archwire or the ease of free tilting of the teeth, particularly the upper incisors. Where such frictional resistance is severe the application of Class II traction can expend lower arch anchorage to very little advantage. In these circumstances application of Class II rubbers can be delayed for a short period, but they should be applied as soon as conditions permit. The light gauge archwires should carry molar anchorage bends and/or tie back stops placed against the molar tubes. The anchor bends alone, however, will be sufficient insurance against the mesial drift of the posterior teeth in most instances.

If multistrand (Twistflex) archwires are employed for preliminary tooth alignment it should be realized that their very flexibility makes them unsuitable for the control of posterior anchorage and, consequently, they should only be used over a very short period and never in association with intermaxillary elastics. Even light 0·014 in or Nitinol archwires should be replaced as soon as their purpose has been served.

First Stage Archwires

Apart from the few occasions, as mentioned above, when some initial alignment of gross tooth malposition is indicated, first stage archwires are made from 0·016 in heat-treated high-tensile

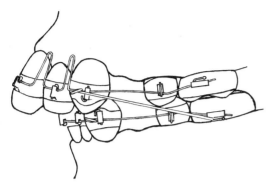

Fig. 3.1. Example of first stage archwires in position on a Class II division 1 malocclusion, from which first bicuspids have been extracted.

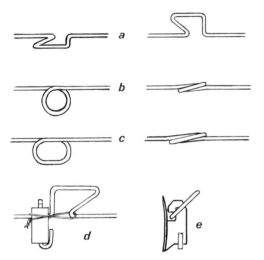

Fig. 3.2. Modes of suspension of inter-maxillary elastics to the main archwire. a, The hook pattern, viewed laterally and from the occlusal. b and c, The round and oval ring patterns, similarly viewed. d, The method of ligation of the inter-maxillary hook to maintain the intercuspid distance and so prevent the advent of spacing. The ligatures must not interfere with freedom of the cuspids to tilt, or, by premature placement, deny the space needed for incisor alignment. e, The angulation of the hook to the buccal in order to prevent the distal arm from becoming locked in the vertical clot of the bracket, thus preventing free tilt.

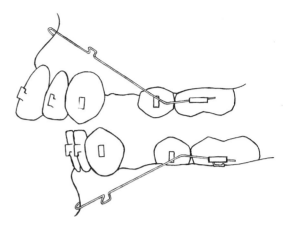

Fig. 3.3. The appearance of Stage 1 and 2 archwires, before pinning. The force values should be assessed by measuring the pressure delivered when the anterior of the archwire is brought to the mouths of the incisor brackets, per individual, and not by the arbitrary use of anchor bends always angled to a standard number of degrees.

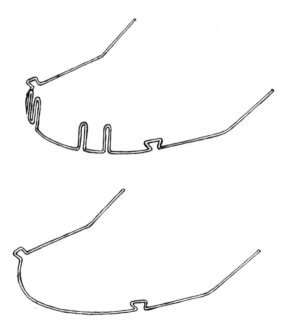

Fig. 3.4. Examples of plain and looped Stage 1 upper archwires. The same forms of archwire are used when inverted, for the lower dental arch.

stainless-steel wire. The qualities exhibited by the wire are important. Much research has been applied to attain qualities of flexibility so that light forces can be developed over the largest deflection of the wire possible. Although this quality is obviously valuable, it is of secondary importance to that of durability against distortion. Force application can always be adjusted, but if inter-bracket spans are too easily distorted so that accidental bends are introduced, the all important control of anchorage may be adversely affected.

The first stage archwires may incorporate anchor bends, toe-in or toe-out bends, vertical

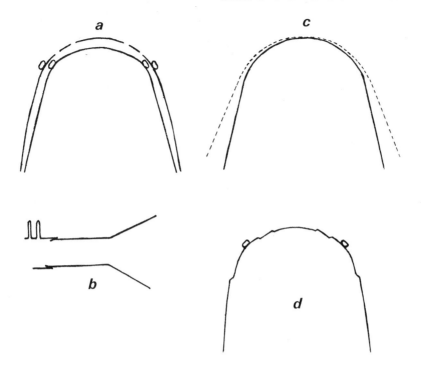

Fig. 3.5. *a* and *b*, Stage 1 archwires, viewed laterally and from the occlusal. *c*, Method of imparting general posterior arch expansion. *d*, Incorporation of bayonet bends and/or premolar offsets.

loops, offset or bayonet bends and inter- or intra-maxillary hooks or coils (*Figs.* 3.1–3.5).

Inter- and Intra-Maxillary Hooks or Coils

These are routinely bent into the archwires for both upper and lower dental arches and are positioned 1 mm to the mesial of the cuspid brackets. The coil pattern of an inter-maxillary hook can be either round or oval and is wound in the same plane as the archwire. If the Z-shaped loop is preferred, the hooks are usually angled somewhat to the buccal, away from the vertical, in order to avoid any possibility of the distal arm of the loop becoming wedged in the slot of the cuspid bracket and so preventing the freedom of that tooth to tilt, thus increasing resistance by introducing bodily movement. Whatever the pattern of inter-maxillary hook employed, the hook must offer the patient ease of application of the rubbers. No justifiable excuse must ever be offered which might induce a failure to wear these vitally important elastics (*Fig.* 3.2).

The 1 mm clearance between the inter-maxillary hooks and the cuspid brackets offers the practical advantage of allowing the archwire, when pinned to the anteriors, to be moved manually left and right in order to determine the presence of any bracket binding. This test cannot be applied if the hooks and brackets are in contact.

When the ring pattern inter-maxillary hooks are used care must be taken that the archwire curvature is maintained, particularly immediately mesial and distal to the hooks. It will be difficult to work in the arch curvature with the fingers in these areas and some work with pliers will be needed. There is also a tendency for the rings to open, or unwind, so upsetting the conformation of the archwire. The Z-shaped hooks do not have this tendency but have the disadvantage of being perhaps more difficult and time consuming to bend.

Molar Anchorage Bends

These are placed immediately posterior to the second bicuspid bracket. They are bent in the opposite plane to that of the archwire, so that when inserted into the buccal tubes the anterior section of the archwires will lie into the buccal sulci before pinning. The amount of bend to be incorporated will be subject to slight variation with each case, rather than determined by any rigid rule, in order that the same force application is produced in each instance (*Fig.* 3.3).

The leverage force on the molars can be assessed by measuring the reciprocal action which intends intrusion of the incisors. If the anterior section of the archwire is brought to, but not into, the opening of the anterior bracket slots, the force should measure about 65 g. Greater forces tend, eventually, to cause undue lingual rolling and distal tilting of the molars and, reciprocally, undue looseness and soreness of the anterior teeth, notably the lower incisors.

It is symptomatic of the use of excess leverage through anchor bends that the mesial marginal ridge of the molars is seen to rise above the occlusal level of the other teeth of the arch. This event should not be awaited with the intention of reducing forces only when it has become apparent because, by then, it is indicative that the mistake has already been made.

Another, none too reliable, test for excess force from the anchor bends is through the behaviour of the archwire in this region as it is placed into the incisor bracket slots. If the force is excessive the bends tend to roll bucally, becoming in this way more a toe-in than an anchor bend, consequently causing the molars to rotate, whilst reducing molar anchorage value.

As the teeth respond the degree of anchor bend may need to be altered to maintain the pressure at a constant level. The test for the correct force value should continue to be applied.

The purpose of the anchor bends in the upper arch is to prevent mesial migration of the upper molars, whilst in the lower arch it is to supply bodily control to the lower molars as these are moved forward by the action of the Class II elastics.

Toe-in Bends

These bends are incorporated into the archwire at the same point as the anchor bends and their purpose is anti-rotational. For example, the lower molars would tend to rotate mesio—lingually under the influence of the inter-maxillary elastics applied to their buccal aspects.

In the design of standard archwires the amount of toe-in will be so slight as to be barely perceptible and never exceed 5°.

In fact, even on light activation, the anchor bends will tend to rotate imperceptibly in the buccal tubes, supplying anti-rotational control almost automatically, without the need for deliberate adjustment.

When the lower archwire is in position and engaged in the anterior brackets, it should emerge from the mesial of the buccal tubes, between 12 and 2 o'clock on the left and 12 and 10 o'clock on the right. The upper archwire should emerge between 6 and 4 o'clock on the left and 6 and 8 o'clock on the right, when the anterior lumen of the tube is taken to represent a clock face.

Toe-out Bends

These supply anti-rotational control in the opposite direction to the toe-in bend, a need which might arise, for example, when using elastic ligatures for local molar or bicuspid rotation. The amount of toe-in or toe-out bend employed in the varied circumstances of treatment is very much a matter for individual operators and can be modified to suit their personal experience. This means, particularly with reference to force values, that orthodontists vary and in consequence have an equally varied need for compensatory mechanisms of which toe-in and toe-out bends are examples. Many orthodontists find no requirement for either during the first stage of treatment.

Toe-in and toe-out bends are not suitable for the correction of severe rotations, but should be used more to prevent rotation than to correct it.

Vertical Loops

These can be used to supply local increased archwire flexibility, or used for space opening or closing, stops, rotation or root torque (*Fig.* 3.6).

It is important to check that any loops employed act only in the way intended and not inadvertantly for one of their other purposes. Only the root torquing loop should overlie and contact the tooth surface. When used otherwise, loops should lie opposite the embrasures between the teeth in such positions that they do not contact the tooth or gingival surfaces, nor protrude unduly towards the cheek or lip, when the archwires are pinned into position.

The loops used for increasing local archwire flexibility are made to a standard size, having a height of 6 mm.

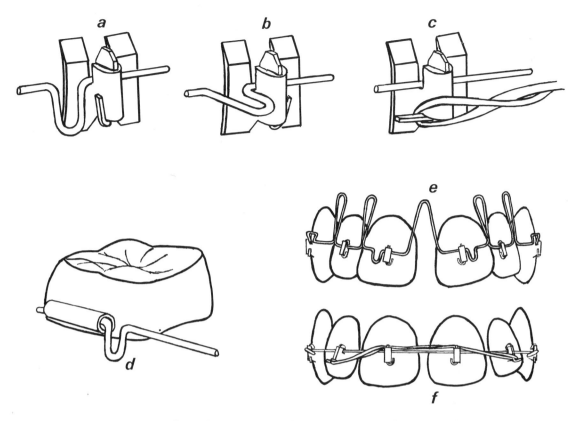

Fig. 3.6. *a, b,* and *d,* Examples of archwire stop loops. Such loops must not interfere with the freedom for the teeth to tilt bucco–lingually, e.g. the retraction of an upper labial segment. *c* and *f,* Use of pin tag as hook for the application of elastic ligatures to effect space closure. *e,* Use of a looped archwire to align incisors and close central diastema.

The trapeze section formed between two vertical loops provides not only additional local flexibility but can, where deemed advisable, be offset from the main line of the archwire to over-rotate or over-correct.

It is not good practice to expand loops to create space for imbricated incisors because this will automatically cause an increase of the inter-cuspid width. Space should be obtained by distal movement of the cuspids which, when Class II traction is employed, will occur spontaneously in the upper arch. Lower cuspids may need individual retraction by very light inter-maxillary elastics if initially they show marked mesial displacement.

In Class II division 1 cases, where the upper laterals are misplaced palatally in association with lack of space, it is often unnecessary to use loops for the purpose of bringing them labially into the line of the arch, but to leave the laterals out of archwire engagement whilst the upper cuspids and centrals are retracted to a point where eventually the laterals can be easily engaged.

Looped archwires used to obtain general alignment should be discarded in favour of plain archwires as soon as the latter can be engaged in the bracket slots with reasonable ease and the avoidance of undue local pressure.

Vertical Loops used for Root Torque

Vertical loops used for root torque will be described later when dealing with the phase of treatment where they are usually employed i.e. at Stage 3 (see Chapter 5). These loops function through contact with the tooth surface and it is of importance to observe that other loops, such as those for additional archwire flexibility, do not contact the tooth or threaten to do so. If this should inadvertently happen, root torque or bodily control will be introduced with possible attendant increased expenditure of anchorage.

Stop Loops

Stop loops or lugs are not usually features of the standard Stage 1 archwires, but there will be occasions where they may have to be incorporated to maintain arch length, to retain the position of a tooth recently repositioned and liable to relapse, or to assist in the transference to the bracket of forces derived from larger space opening or closing loops (*Fig. 3.6e*).

Loops for these purposes will be approximately one third the size of loops used for active force production. As with the torque loops or spurs, so with stop loops; care must be taken that they do not inadvertently interfere with the free tilting of teeth and introduce bodily control where it is not required. For example, if stop loops are bent at right angles to the plane of an upper archwire in a gingival direction and applied to one or more upper incisors which are being retracted to reduce overjet, bodily control will be brought about as soon as the upper incisors have tilted sufficiently to bring the loops into contact with their labial surfaces.

Where the incisors are to be retracted palatally, the stop loops must be either on the incisal side of the archwire or placed in the same plane as the main arch, if the above form of interference is to be avoided (*Fig. 3.6a, b*).

Bayonet Bends

It is inadvisable to use bayonet bends for active correction, because of the tendency for round archwires to rotate within the bracket slots, causing the bayonet bend to become ineffective, or even to supply movement in the wrong plane.

The bayonet bend has been commonly used passively to retain over-rotation brought about via a previous looped arch (*Fig. 3.5d*). This practice is becoming less popular as more operators advise against the need to over-correct rotations when using full fixed apparatus.

If and when bayonet bends are incorporated into archwire design for the above purpose they should be small, the offset section being some 5° to the line of the main arch. All such bends should be of the same standard size.

Bicuspid Offsets

In most instances the first stage archwires, when viewed from the occlusal, can be kept straight from the distal of the cuspids to the ends of the wire with no offset bends.

There are occasions, however, when it will be found that a plain archwire of this type bears against the brackets of the second bicupsids, even though the molar is not rotated mesio–palatally nor the bicuspid displaced buccally. Broadening the archwire in the inter-cuspid region may appear to overcome the difficulty, but will innevitably produce an undesirable expansion of the dental arch in that region.

The placement of small bicuspid offset bends in the plane of the archwire opposite the centre of the extraction sites and well to the mesial of the second bicuspid brackets in such circumstances, assists the avoidance of inter-cuspid expansion and palatal displacement of the bicuspids. Lingual rolling of the second lower bicuspids as these are moved mesially into a convergent part of the archwire will also be avoided (*Fig. 3.5d*).

Archwire Form, Dimension and Correlation

Since one of the aims of treatment will be to establish arch symmetry, the archwires themselves will be made symmetrical. The objective is to correct the malocclusion, not to preserve defects.

To this end, the anterior section of the archwires, from the distal of the cuspid on the one side to the distal of that on the other, is formed into a symmetrical smooth curve. The curve should be suited to the individual and not impart any expansion of the inter-cuspid width.

From the distal of the cuspid to the molar the archwire is kept straight, with the possible exceptions of very slight toe-in of the anchor bend section distal to the second bicuspid bracket and of premolar offsets when included.

If the archwire design incorporates vertical loops or other forms of adjustment bends these must not be allowed to upset the general archwire symmetry, when viewed from the occlusal, (*Fig. 3.5a*).

Looked at in the opposite plane, the whole of the archwire, inclusive of any sections between loops, should lie flat against any flat surface, with the exception of the regions posterior to the anchor bends (*Fig. 3.5b*).

When the upper and lower archwires have been made, they need to be correlated to avoid un-intentional contraction or expansion which might result in crossbite production. To this end the original study casts should be consulted for general arch form and cuspid and molar widths. It is help-ful if these dimensions are transferred to graph paper and an ideal arch diagram created which can be referred to throughout treatment.

Unless care is taken over arch dimensions it is easy to expand fractionally with each successive archwire, resulting, by the completion of treat-ment, in considerable arch enlargement which may not remain stable. A lack of correlation can be introduced with detrimental results when one archwire is changed—because, for example, it has become damaged—but not the other. The availability of an ideal archwire diagram can materially assist continued correlation.

After symmetrical construction and arch coordination a further adjustment is required for each archwire.

Both archwires, in the treatment of Class II division 1 on the standard three stage principles of the Begg technique, are kept expanded across the molar region. The lower archwire is expanded a total of 1 cm, evenly distributed to both sides. The upper archwire is also kept expanded, but by only half the amount, i.e. 5 mm.

The above requirements do not imply expansion in the cuspid region. The expansion is applied to the archwires distal to the cuspid brackets by slight decrease of the anterior curvature. Once placed in the buccal tubes the anterior curvature is restored, and the wire should slip passively into the cuspid bracket slots (Fig. 3.5c).

Keeping the archwires expanded posteriorly in the above manner should not produce actual expansion. It is a compensatory mechanism, counteracting a contraction across the molar region which would otherwise occur.

If cuspids are rotated, the angle of their bracket slots in the horizontal plane will be affected so that the distal ends of the archwire will be thrown out, or in, as soon as it is seated in the slots. This factor must be taken into consideration when establishing the relationship of the distal ends of the archwire to the molars. Because of this factor, combined with that of friction when dealing with marked cuspid rotation, particularly in the upper arch, it may be advisable to eliminate the worst of the discrepancy as a separate stage at the outset

of treatment, even if it means extending the overall period of active intervention.

Pins, Pinning and Ligation of Archwires

It is important before placing the archwires to establish that the bracket slots are open, so that there will be no obstruction to the freedom of the wire to slide, and that the pin channels are free of cement plugs.

The modern brackets are stronger than some of their forebears but, even so, their slots should be checked to see that they have not become partially occluded by distortion during band cementation or from other causes.

The lock pins used must be those designed for the particular make of bracket that has been fitted. The pins used during the opening stages of treatment should be of the safety lock design which automatically obviate friction between pin head and archwire.

In the first stage of the treatment of Class II malocclusion all teeth are pinned, with the follow-ing exceptions:

(1) The second bicuspids.
(2) Teeth initially so far displaced, either in the horizontal or vertical direction, that they cannot be reached by the archwire, or, if they can be so reached, excessive force application results.
(3) Upper lateral incisors which are lingual to the centrals in Class II division 1 occlusions, and nearly correctly related to the lower incisors.
(4) Rotated buccal teeth, where the bracket has been deliberately offset so that the archwire cannot be seated fully into the bracket slot until the rotation has been rectified, or where the full bracket engage-ment of the archwire would actually prevent correction of rotation.

In situation (2) above, the brackets of the displaced teeth are ligated to the archwire to gain initial movement and to bring the bracket slots progressively to the point where pinning becomes possible without generating undue pressure at any time during the full correction. A looped archwire may be of advantage in gaining increased deflection whilst maintaining the important lightness of pressure where this is not possible using a plain arch. The same procedure can be adopted in situation (4): the span of archwire between

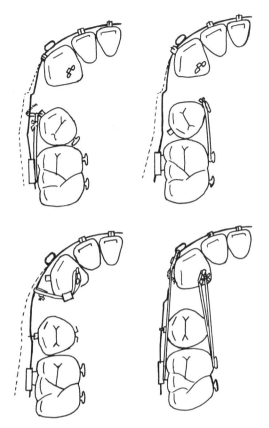

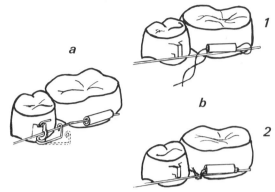

Fig. 3.8. a, Method of promoting local tooth rotation by spring auxiliary. b 1 and 2, Method of applying a ligature to rotate a molar, when access to the mesial opening of the tube by the archwire is obstructed.

Fig. 3.7. Some examples of elastic ligature ties to effect various rotations. Anti-rotational control of the molars is supplied through toe-in or toe-out bends, whichever is appropriate to counter the direction of the reciprocal force. Once the rotated teeth have been corrected, the elastic ligatures can be replaced by steel ligatures. The brackets of the rotated teeth can be slightly offset, so that they will be held in mildly overcorrected positions when finally engaged with the main archwire.

vertical loops is engaged in the bracket slot as early as possible to gain positive control over the rotation. Force application is kept light even if in the case of severe rotation, the inter-loop span has actually to be offset in the direction of the rotation, being thereafter periodically adjusted to complete the movement by degrees. Where rotation is being corrected by elastic ligature or spring auxiliary, the archwire is kept outside the bracket slot to avoid obstructing the movement (*see* rotation methods, *Figs.* 3.7 and 3.8).

In situation (3) it is frequently pointless to move the lateral incisors labially into line with the centrals for the sake of the privilege of retracting them to their original position. If the lateral incisors occupy a reasonably good relationship to the lowers they can be left unbanded until the centrals and cuspids have been retracted to reduce overjet. As this is done the archwire will get closer to the laterals so that their brackets can eventually be engaged.

Situation (1) refers to the first bicuspid extraction case. The second bicuspids are never pinned during the first stage of treatment for such a case whilst the extraction sites remain open. Instead the archwire is designed to bypass the second bicuspid brackets buccally. The archwire should be in near contact with the brackets, unless the teeth are lingually displaced. In order to protect the archwire against damage, to assist the vertical orientation of the second bicuspids where needed and to give increased stability to the posterior anchor bends, the wire is held to the bracket with a bypass clamp (*Fig.* 3.1). This method of supporting the archwire is preferable to the use of steel ligatures for the same purpose. If the latter are used they must not be tied so tightly as to cause frictional resistance to the sliding of the wire. The ligature, or bypass clamp, should be mesial to the molar anchor bend.

It must be seen that the support given to the archwires by the bypass clamps or ligatures does not interfere with or eliminate the depression force to the anteriors. This should seldom happen if the anchor bends are correctly located. Should it occur even in these circumstances, the second bicuspids can be left unattached to the archwire or, if attachment is retained, further bends introduced to continue incisor depression. This would mean, in the upper arch, the curving of the archwire to give an increased curve of Spee and, in the lower arch, the opposite, or reverse curvature.

The free ends, or tags, of the locking pins should be routinely turned around the brackets in a mesial direction. This ensures that the ends of the pins do not contact the archwire should the teeth tilt distally, which in the case of the anteriors is their usual direction. The knowledge that the tags have been turned to the mesial will eliminate confusion when unpinning.

Frictional resistance will occur if the tags contact the archwire, but it should be noted that they are nevertheless turned well round the bracket. It is tempting to save a few seconds chairside time by turning the pin tags through no more than 90°, or even less. The pins are made of soft brass and, if not turned firmly round the brackets, can reopen releasing the archwire with variable consequences, some of which can make nonsense of the original object of time saving.

When using a steel ligature instead of a pin for firm ligation, the ligature wire is first passed through the vertical channel of the bracket, its gingival end passing on the tooth side of the archwire. This end is then brought over the archwire and passed out to the mesial or distal of the archwire slot. The archwire will not be held firmly if the ligature is passed out of the top and bottom of the pin channel. (see Chapter 2 Fig. 2.1).

In addition to pinning and ligation as described above, further ligatures may be needed. If incisor teeth threaten to become spaced, the inter-maxillary hooks are tied to the main archwire immediately distal to the cuspid brackets. The measure prevents any further independent distal movement of the cuspids, which in turn assures that the inter-cuspid distance is maintained. These ligatures must pass over the buccal of the cuspid brackets and not around the top or bottom, which might interfere with the free tilting of the cuspids (Fig. 3.2d). If small single module elastic rings are used instead of ligatures for the above purpose, they too must pass over the buccal of the cuspid brackets and not be so tight that free tilting is threatened. The elastic rings must be slipped over the ends of the archwire before insertion into the buccal tubes.

No ties of this kind should be placed when incisors are crowded because by maintaining the inter-cuspid distance the opening of the necessary space will be prevented.

If the inter-maxillary hook ligatures are not applied early enough to prevent incisor spacing, the space can be closed either by re-introducing a looped arch or by elastic ligature. The tags of the lock pins can be used as hooks, suitably angled, to support elastics or elastic ligatures (Fig. 3.6c).

Buccal Tubes and Archwire Sliding

In order that the upper and lower archwires can slide freely, the wire should protrude a short distance from the distal of the buccal tubes and not be lodged within them. The wire must not protrude so as to contact the gingival tissues or the mesial of the second permanent molar.

As treatment proceeds, the positions of both the anchor bends and the ends of the archwires must be checked on every occasion of inspection. When the upper anteriors are retracted and, at the same time, the lower posteriors are moved mesially, the anchor bends get progressively closer to the entrance to the buccal tubes with ever increasing frictional resistance, upsetting progress and force distribution. Adjustment, or new archwires, will be needed to overcome this. At the same time the wire must be adjusted to the shortening arch length so that excess wire distal to the buccal tubes is eliminated before causing damage or preventing continued movement.

Inter- and Intra-Maxillary Elastics

In considering the use of Class II inter-maxillary elastics, note should be taken of the nature of mechanical, control given to the teeth at either end of the elastic action.

Bodily control of the lower molars is provided through the interaction of archwire and buccal tube. The archwire is, however, of small gauge whilst the tube is relatively large. The effect of combining these facts with the further facts that both wire and tubes are round and that the second bicuspids are only loosely held to the archwire by a bypass clamp and are not firmly held by bracket engagement, is to produce a mechanical control that is both tenuous and flimsy. Molar anchorage control thus delicately held can easily be overcome by all but the lightest of elastic forces.

If the force applied exceeds the maximum recommended 70 g for each side, the result may be that the anchor teeth will suffer undue elevation, lingual rolling, rotation and general mesial and lingual displacement, accompanied by possible soreness and looseness.

At the other end of the elastic pull, the upper anteriors are permitted to tilt freely. Only under conditions of really light forces will the apices of these teeth remain relatively undisturbed, showing only a slight movement labially. The usual recommended range for the inter-maxillary elastic force is 60–70 g, although a very acceptable rate of response can be expected in many patients with even less pressure when the elastics are worn, as they should be, continuously. The more the maximum recommended force is exceeded, the greater the probability that the rate of movement of the upper incisor root apices labially equals or exceeds the rate of movement of the crown palatally. Over a given period of treatment, this would mean that the upper incisors reach a vertical or palatally inclined position earlier than necessary relative to the amount of overjet reduction achieved in the same period. The same circumstances also imply that the upper incisor roots may be brought firmly into contact with the labial cortical plate and, if heavy pressure continues to be maintained, loss of apical tooth tissue may result.

The ease with which free tilting of the upper incisors would seem to permit reduction of overjet brings with it the temptation to break speed records in this respect by employing forces which are greater than those that either the teeth or the mechanics of the appliance will tolerate. The temptation must be overcome if treatment standards are not to suffer from the build up of one undesirable side effect upon another.

Some orthodontists have led themselves to believe that excess inter-maxillary forces can be used so long as compensation is afforded by increasing the molar anchorage bends to supply the resistance. It is true that the anchor bend forces and those of the inter-maxillary elastics should be coordinated, but only when the forces are kept to the proper level will the results be advantageous. Excess forces from the anchor bends produce their own chain of detrimental effects, e.g. excessive distal tipping of the lower molars, often with associated resorption of the roots, particularly the mesial, and an increased liability to lingual rolling and contraction of the inter-molar width. As the molars tilt distally so do the buccal tubes, resulting in the anchor bends themselves rising occlusally, thus becoming more liable to damage, with further adverse consequences.

For the same reasons as above, intra-maxillary or Class III elastic forces, when used, should be kept within the 70 g limit; indeed in many instances, half that amount may prove sufficient for consistent improvement.

No comparison should be permitted between the force values employed in the Begg technique and those of edgewise or other fixed appliance which utilize brackets slotted in the same plane as the archwire. The edgewise type of bracket prevents mesio–distal tipping and, consequently, this prevention produces frictional resistance when teeth are moved mesio–distally. Such resistance will need to be overcome, demanding force applications higher than those either necessary or advisable with the Begg apparatus. The axial control given by the edgewise bracket and rectangular archwire is three dimensionally complete, so that the higher forces do not produce the detrimental results which they might with the Begg bracket/archwire liaison.

The light force application with the Begg appliance is, therefore, a practical requirement, to which arguments on theoretical benefit or otherwise of so-called pathological or physiological pressures are quite incidental. The inter-maxillary elastics (Class II) are applied to the archwire hooks mesial to the upper cuspids and over the buccal hooks on the lower molars. Alternatively they can be placed over hooks, buttons, or cleats on the lingual aspect of the lower molars, to help combat situations where the lower molars tend to roll lingually.

The force delivered by an inter-maxillary elastic should be measured by a suitable instrument. The instruments usually available for the purpose are not renowned for their accuracy, but at least they provide a better assessment than arbitrary judgement. After applying the rubber to the molar hook, the force is measured at the cuspid hook when the teeth are in occlusion. The reading will give the minimal force value, which will rise when the patient opens the mouth.

Objectives of the First Stage of Treatment

The first sets of archwires will complete general alignment of the teeth, reduce overbite to an edge-to-edge incisor relationship and correct the relationship of the posterior teeth, upper to lower, where such is required.

These objectives must be completed before embarking on the next stage of treatment. Keeping the three stages of treatment completely separate is a sound basic rule, particularly for those least experienced with the Begg appliance and technique. It must be admitted however, that it is difficult to find any rule applicable to any form of appliance therapy which is universally suited to every circumstance of treatment, even within a given stage. It will be seen later that there are occasions when elements of one stage may become associated with elements of another.

The means by which the teeth are brought into alignment using one or more sets of archwires should already be apparent, since the methods used do not differ in principle from those used by many other appliances and are dependent on archwire flexibility and the balance of anchorage between units or a group of units.

Overbite reduction is brought about by the reciprocal action of the molar anchorage bends as they produce their intrusive force anteriorly. The vertical component of force from the inter-maxillary elastics assists elevation of the lower molars, so aiding the depressive forces on the lower incisors, but equally reducing the intrusive effect on the upper anteriors.

The inter-maxillary elastics supply the horizontal component of force which retracts the upper anteriors, reducing overjet whilst bringing forward the lower posteriors into the extraction sites and into a Class I relationship with the uppers.

The direct function of the molar anchor bends is to supply, in the upper arch, gentle distal leverage to the molars to prevent their mesial migration during treatment, whilst, in the lower arch, the same distal leverage, balanced with the inter-maxillary force, should cause the lower molars to move forward bodily, showing no tilt to the mesial or distal.

This bodily control over the lower molars against the pull of the inter-maxillary elastics, is the main source of anchorage during Stage 1. The fact that the upper anteriors are allowed to tip freely at the opposite end of the elastic pull, provides a free tilt versus bodily movement balance, which is the first contribution towards the important feature of anchorage economy offered by the Begg appliance.

At the conclusion of the first stage of treatment there may be residual space in the extraction sites, varying in amount with the original degree of overcrowding and the success or otherwise of anchorage conservation accompanying treatment thus far.

The space left in the extraction sites may be evenly or unevenly distributed. The action to be taken in respect to the residual space is the concern of the next, or second stage of treatment.

Additional Items of Relevance to Stage 1

Before describing the procedures of Stage 2 of treatment, one or two items remain which should be added to the description of Stage 1.

Correction of Buccal Crossbite

Crossbites, whether buccal or anterior, often have a strong underlying skeletal element. In the case of buccal crossbite an arch width discrepancy may be the fundamental cause rather than tooth displacement. Some such crossbites, where the skeleton rather than the teeth is at fault, may not be correctable by orthodontic appliance. In some such instances, the teeth may be already angled in such a way as to compensate for the arch width discrepancy, as far as is possible; in others the crossbite has been present for a long time, possibly even in the deciduous dentition. In these latter cases, often Class III occlusions, there has sometimes been an early limited period of unilateral condylar growth which can help the patient to establish permanently what had previously been a bite of convenience. The result is, in the long run, a mild facial asymmetry in association with the buccal crossbite and no mandibular deviation on closure, i.e. as a result of one time uneven condylar growth the mandible is swung to left or right. On closure the teeth are brought directly into a functional, but technically incorrect relationship. It may be impossible to compensate for such discrepancies through orthodontic tooth movement.

Where buccal crossbite has resulted from local tooth displacement or angulation, correction can be achieved, as in other techniques, by the use of cross-elastics worn between the buccal hooks on the lower first permanent molars and buttons, cleats, or a hook on the lingual aspect of the uppers. The movement can be supplemented by springing the main archwires in the appropriate directions.

Rotation

Rotation of the teeth can be carried out by one of three methods, in accordance with patient and mechanical convenience:

(1) Use of the section of archwire between two vertical loops;

(2) Use of elastic ligature, thread or coil spring; or

(3) Use of spring auxiliary fitted to the bracket and latched to the main archwire.

Elimination of rotation amongst teeth is one of the first requirements in treatment. The presence of rotated teeth, particularly if the rotations are severe, can produce local friction between bracket and archwire which, in turn, interferes with the freedom of the archwire to slide and the freedom of the teeth to tilt, thereby possibly upsetting the balance of anchorage when Class II rubbers are applied. As mentioned earlier, it may be wise to reduce the more severe rotations as a preliminary stage of treatment and only introduce the inter-maxillary forces when alignment is complete, or nearly so. The presence of rotated teeth can also upset archwire symmetry and influence the general posterior archwire expansion.

In the worst cases looped archwires with molar stops to maintain arch length can be used, with molar anchor bends much reduced, until the majority of the malalignment has been erased, when standard Stage 1 procedures can be started.

It should be emphasized that the above measures are not necessary when rotation is mild and it is judged that frictional elements, stemming from archwire or elastic ligatures, are insufficient to interfere with the efficiency of the Class II mechanics.

The most convenient method of eliminating rotation in the labial segments is by the use of a looped arch, although, where the cuspids are concerned, elastic ligatures are often preferred. The use of elastic ligatures rather than vertical loops is probably the most convenient and effective method of correcting bicuspid rotation and can sometimes be extended to assist molar rotation.

When the trapeze section between vertical loops is used it should be so adjusted that a light positive force, in the appropriate direction, is applied to the tooth. This means that no great effort should be needed to seat the archwire in the bracket slot. The over-enthusiastic application of force can result both in increased mobility of the affected teeth and in unnecessary pain to the patient.

When elastic ligatures are used for the rotation of cuspids and bicuspids it will be necessary to equip these teeth with either lingual buttons or cleats. The main archwire will be kept out of the bracket slot and clear of the bracket itself, so that there is no impediment to the intended rotation. The brackets are often offset slightly in order to bring about mild over-correction.

Examples of rotatory ties and their compensatory archwire adjustments are shown in *Fig. 3.7*.

Figure 3.8a illustrates a form of auxiliary spring suitable to the correction of rotation. This auxiliary is seldom used as a part of general early tooth alignment, but more often for the correction of an isolated unit in the later phases of treatment.

The choice of rotatory method is at the orthodontist's own discretion, which will depend on his assessment of the total, rather than local, action of the appliance at the particular stage of treatment reached.

Rotated molars are a particular problem which will upset normal operation of the appliance mechanics until corrected. If the molar is rotated mesio—lingually it will be impossible to insert the archwire into the buccal tube, the mesial opening of which will be inaccessible behind the second bicuspid.

If the rotation is mild it may be possible by not fitting the bicuspid bracket to gain access to the buccal tube with the archwire, but when more severe the method shown in *Fig.* 3.8b can be employed. The archwire is outside the tube and held by a steel ligature, first passed through the tube. The wire is held by the distal loop of the ligature emerging from the distal of the tube and the free ends of the ligature are tied round the archwire at the mesial. The rotatory effect, as administered, can usefully be augmented by applying the inter-maxillary elastic to a hook or cleat on the lingual side of the molar.

There will, inevitably, be frictional resistance between archwire and tube when the above method is used. Indeed this is a natural consequence of molar rotation, whether the archwire is inside or outside the tube, or a vertical loop is introduced mesial to the molar to increase local archwire flexibility, or whether a recurved archwire is used

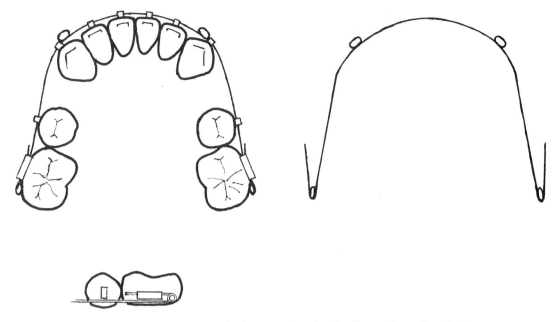

Fig. 3.9. The recurved archwire for correction of molar tilt, rotation or lingual roll.

to cure the rotation (*Fig.* 3.9). It may be safer therefore, as with other rotations, to correct the discrepancy before instituting full Class II mechanics. This is not to say that one can never get away with the combined action. The orthodontist must assess very carefully the possible consequences of any action in situations where frictional binding is involved.

Damage to Archwires

Damage to archwires can be broadly divided into two categories:

(1) Accidental; and

(2) Habitual.

Every effort is made to avoid the possibility of damage to the archwires by keeping the buccal tubes and second bicuspid brackets well to the gingival, so that the vitally important anchor bends are thereby kept as far as possible from the cusps of the teeth of the opposing arch. In areas where no teeth are present which might be used for archwire support the unsupported span is stepped gingivally so as to minimize the risk both of damage from the teeth of the opposite arch and of the use of the archwire for masticatory purposes (*Fig.* 3.10). Archwire gauge will be as

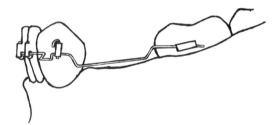

Fig. 3.10. Unsupported section of archwire stepped gingivally to minimize the risk of distortion from occlusal forces. Such action is particularly relevant to the lower arch and still more so in areas of that arch where there happens to be an absence of teeth.

large as is consistant with the role of archwires as agents for tooth movement.

Archwires are at their most vulnerable during Stage 1 when, for reason of required flexibility the smaller gauges of wire have to be used, there are open extraction sites present and the dental arch lengths are at their maximum.

When damage occurs to the archwires it is usually in the inter-bracket spans and can vary in severity. The wires should be removed at the slightest sign of damage, since any bend, accidentally introduced, alters force values and directions.

Even a slight distortion may be seen to be of greater significance than is at first suspected, once the archwire has been removed.

When accidents introduce bad distortions, or the anchor bends are bitten out, the archwires must be immediately replaced. When such accidents are frequent with the same patient, and of severe degree, it could be that he or she is in the habit of crunching hard food, e.g. boiled sweets.

The habitual form of damage arises in the same way and in the same places, but is mild in degree. Slight distortion of the inter-bracket spans may be seen to be repeated by the same patient in the same areas and may be related to cusps of opposing teeth. These small bends can be safely left, so long as the general arch form is not affected and the anchor bends are readjusted to their correct level of force application. Eliminating these habitual bends is of no avail, because they will almost certainly soon be reintroduced.

Difficulty in Obtaining Overbite Reduction

Probably the commonest mechanical reason for failure to fully reduce overbite is inconsistency of patient co-operation in the wearing of inter-maxillary elastics. It is, however, a fact that overbite reduction is greatly assisted by appropriate increases in lower anterior facial height, coincident with the period of active treatment, through growth. Patients who show below-average development in that location during active treatment will provide greater problems in overbite elimination.

These latter patients include those whose mandibular growth follows the closing rotation pattern, the mandible itself often displaying a low gonial angle.

In the case of obdurate overbite reduction the use of additional archwire forces through increase of the anchor bends may well not have the intended effect, but instead produce rolling of the molars, loss of anchorage, apical resorption and increased mobility of both molars and incisors, particularly lowers. These are the same items, already cited, that result from attempts to increase the anchorage value of the lower first permanent molars by increasing the molar anchorage bends excessively in order to counter an equally excessive pull of inter-maxillary elastics.

The molars do not only supply horizontal anchorage but, in the case of overbite reduction, vertical anchorage also. Since, for all practical purposes, in the Begg appliance they are the sole suppliers, it follows that forces deployed to intrude the anterior teeth must also affect the molars. Excess forces produced through the anchor bends may, therefore, not only generate the reactions stated above, but also cause the molars to tilt distally with elevation of the mesial marginal ridge and relative depression of the posterior.

It is consequently helpful if ways can be found of reinforcing the posterior anchorage in the vertical dimension. There are two.

The first is by the use of vertical inter-maxillary elastics suspended between the distal ends of the upper and lower archwires as they protrude from the posterior of the buccal tubes on each side. These cause a general elevation of the posterior teeth and support the distal of the molars, thus reinforcing the depressive force supplied to the anteriors through the archwires. In order that these elastics do not slip off the distal ends of the archwires the latter must be turned towards the gingival to become retaining hooks. When the above system is used it should be borne in mind that an additional load is being placed on the lower molars, which are already supporting the Class II inter-maxillary rubbers.

The second system has seldom been advocated for the Begg appliance, although successful with other types of fixed appliance. The lower first permanent molar can be given support against distal tilt by Banding the second permanent molar when available and carrying the archwire back to those teeth. The system is sound in principle, in that the inclusion of the second molar reinforces available vertical anchorage, but application in the context of the Begg appliance and technique raises a number of technical problems. For example, since the inclusion of the second molars will alter the balance of anchorage in the horizontal dimension as well as the vertical, some suitable means of containing the archwire on the first molar will have to be found and the vertical height orientation of the buccal attachments in general will have to be modified. It could even be found that the most practical form of attachment for the first permanent molar, in the circumstances, would be of an edgewise pattern rather than Begg, which would no doubt greatly upset the purists. Certainly the effectiveness of the appliance would be upset if the standard usage were not to be altered to compensate. At present the second molar is not used in the above manner with the Begg appliance, but the possibility remains.

Full overbite reduction is of the utmost importance to the whole quality of treatment results, for without it, the proper relationship of the buccal teeth cannot be achieved. Further detailed reference to the overbite problem will be made later in the text.

Patient Cooperation, Care and Maintainance of the Appliance

Every orthodontist will develop his own opinions on the importance of, and the method by which, he puts his patient in the picture and obtains the requisite standards of cooperation.

It might be helpful, nevertheless, to suggest that instruction to the patient might be divided between matters concerning the care of the appliance, involving instruction in the best forms of oral hygiene, and the matter of the importance of the inter-maxillary elastics.

The latter, supplying perhaps 60% of the action in tooth movement, is so vital as to be worthy of being presented as a separate issue. Many patients are seemingly impressed with the complexity of the archwires, bands, brackets and auxiliaries, but remain so unimpressed by ordinary elastic bands that they assume that the latter are not really necessary. Some form of sales talk is indicated, perhaps likening the elastics to the engine of a machine and the remainder of the appliance to the brakes, steering, gears etc. However the matter is put, the instruction must be imparted with a clear indication of its importance and not linked to other, perhaps to many rather boring, instructions which might tend to cloud the issue.

The inter-maxillary elastics should be worn continuously and changed every three to five days. Should a breakage of one occur, it is probably advisable for the patient not only to replace it, but also to replace the one on the opposite side.

This ensures that the force application continues the same bilaterally.

The frequency of attendance for appliance adjustment and progress assessment is a matter for the individual orthodontist to determine.

In general terms, it can be said that Stage 1 demands more intense supervision than the later stages of treatment for the following reasons:

(1) The patient is new to appliance experience;
(2) The patient's capacity to cooperate is still to become known to the orthodontist;
(3) The extraction sites are open and the individual teeth in positions of maximum disorder, so that there are possibly long spans of unsupported archwire and some teeth which cannot initially be pinned, leading to a general vulnerability of the apparatus as a whole;
(4) The need for archwire flexibility dictates that the lightest gauges of wire are used which also implies relative vulnerability to damage, and more so when it is realized that the archwires are at their longest at the outset of treatment of an extraction case.
(5) There is a large amount of simultaneous mechanical action taking place in association with the general appliance vulnerability.

Any serious mistake made during Stage 1 may well not be fully recoverable later. In order to keep a strict eye on the appliance and progress, the period between visits for the purpose should be about a month.

Later, as spaces are closed, teeth well aligned and fully pinned, larger gauge archwires employed and the problems set out above eliminated, the interval between each visit can be extended at the orthodontist's discretion.

For all its complexity, Stage 3 of treatment probably needs the least supervision, so long as the initial mechanical assembly of the multiple parts has been properly and securely carried out. Six-week intervals should suffice during Stage 3.

Chapter 4

Objectives and mechanics of the second phase of treatment (Stage 2)

The purpose of the second stage of treatment is usually described, with maximum brevity, as the closure of space in the extraction sites. This can be regarded as an oversimplification of the facts and spacing should not be closed arbitrarily, without prior thought and assessment.

The following points should be considered when proceeding to Stage 2:

(1) That the objectives of Stage 1 have been fully reached;

(2) That the anchorage claims of the mechanics of the next and final stage of treatment (Stage 3) have been worked out in theory;

(3) That consideration has been given to the timing of centre line correction, if such be needed, whilst space still remains for its accomplishment;

(4) That, in respect of the correction of any marked centre line discrepancy, it has been previously noted that there will be a separate space closure stage. It can happen that the amount and rate of tooth movement in Stage 1 results in the extraction sites becoming closed at a time coincident with the completion of Stage 1 objectives;

(5) That, as a result of general alignment carried out in Stage 1, it is now easier to determine any fault in band or bracket positioning. These should be rectified before the commencement of Stage 3 and whilst the appliance mechanics remain relatively simple; and

(6) That any spacing amongst the anteriors has been closed.

The Mechanics of Stage 2

Archwires

The archwire pattern is basically that of the first stage of treatment. 0·016 in gauge of wire can still be used, although some orthodontists now prefer 0·018 in or 0·020 in in order to obtain full alignment of the anterior segments and give more rigidity to the appliance with increased resistance to damage. In those instances where there has been frequent archwire distortion or unilateral space closure, the larger gauge has obvious advantage, but in most cases the change can be regarded as optional. Whatever the gauge of archwire chosen, anchor bends coupled with minimal toe-in are incorporated, as in Stage 1, immediately posterior to the second bicuspid bracket. The pressure supplied by the anchor bends to molars and incisors is slightly reduced from that employed during Stage 1.

The archwires should be symmetrical and will have been correlated upper to lower. Both are kept expanded in the molar regions, as in Stage 1, but the amount of expansion will be slightly reduced, unless clinical analysis at this point decrees otherwise. When placed in the molar tubes, the archwires should engage the cuspid brackets passively and not encourage inter-cuspid expansion.

Inter-maxillary hooks are incorporated in both archwires immediately mesial to the cuspid brackets and in contact, or very near contact, with them. The hooks in the upper arch often have to contain two elastics each during Stage 2, which is sometimes difficult with the ring pattern. A Z-shaped hook makes it easier for the patient to apply two rubbers to the same hook. Whichever pattern is used, it must be said that the patient should not be at any time provided with an enforced excuse for non-cooperation. If the inter-maxillary hooks, either anterior or posterior, are difficult to access, or inadequate, the patient will soon cease to apply the elastics and this temporary luxury may make it difficult for him to return to the correct regimen.

If the Z-loops are employed the distal limb

must not be able to enter the slot of the cuspid bracket, since this could produce bodily control over the cuspid. By placing these hooks at an angle to the plane of the archwire in a buccal direction the possible occurrence will be prevented.

Small bicuspid offsets can be included in either archwire, distal to the cuspids and sufficiently mesial to the second bicuspid brackets, to allow the latter to move towards closure with the cuspids, without being displaced lingually. There is no need for the offsets where such displacement is not threatened.

The former practice of incorporating bayonet bends to hold teeth that have been rotated, in over-corrected positions, has not been found to be notably advantageous and many orthodontists now prefer plain archwires.

The archwires once completed, checked for symmetry and correlation, are pinned to the upper and lower six anteriors. The second bicuspids are bypassed as in Stage 1, the wire lying on the buccal surface of the brackets and held in position by bypass clamp, or steel ligature.

Stage 2 should not be carried out without the second bicuspids being held to the archwire as, should overclosure of the extraction sites unintentionally occur, the unattached teeth may be squeezed out of the line of the arch and so give difficulty and unnecessary time loss in their recovery. The use of bands and brackets at this stage, should they not have been fitted earlier, will not only prevent the bicuspids from becoming displaced lingually, but also assist their orientation in the vertical plane, so making full bracket engagement, when the time comes, that much the easier.

The inter-maxillary hooks, in each arch, are ligated to the main archwire immediately distal to the cuspid brackets, in the same manner as in Stage 1, to hold the anteriors together as a unit.

Use of Inter- and Intra-Maxillary Elastics in Stage 2

These elastics supply the motive forces for the tooth movements that are to result in the elimination of residual space in the extraction sites.

At or near the commencement of Stage 2 is a suitable time to obtain a lateral skull radiograph from which to assess treatment progress, whilst space in the extraction sites still remains. From the radiograph, using cephalometric measurements, the antero—posterior positions of the labial segments can be determined and compared to their positions shown on the original radiograph, taken at the commencement of active treatment.

It will be seen from this comparison whether space should be closed through further retraction of the labial segments or by movement of the posterior segments in the opposite direction. If both these measures are needed in some degree, the balance of reciprocal movement can be determined and the mechanics adjusted accordingly. Once space has been closed, room for this important manoeuvre will have been lost.

In determining the balance of mechanical action for this stage, clinical judgement with cephalometric support are taken into consideration with an assessment of anchorage response, not only for the remainder of Stage 2 but also for Stage 3 of treatment.

In Stage 3 the positions of the apices of the teeth are corrected, resulting in the proper orientation of the long axes of their roots.

In the typical Class II division 1 case, where first bicuspids have been extracted, the usual requirements for Stage 3 are that the cuspid apices be moved distally, the second bicuspid apices mesially and the upper central incisor roots torqued palatally. The upper lateral incisors may require either palatal or labial apical torque as well as needing their apices to be moved distally. The distal movement of apices also applies to the lower laterals in most instances.

When the root apex of a tooth is moved by mechanical force, the crown of that tooth will move in the opposite direction unless restrained. Because of this factor there will be a balance of reciprocal apical anchorage set up by the root movements of Stage 3.

In the Class II example just given the number and root area of the teeth requiring distal or palatal apical movement exceeds those demanding the opposite action. The result will be a slight general shift of the crowns of the teeth of both arches towards the anterior, which will gradually take place during Stage 3. The incisor crowns, therefore, will be moved towards the lips.

It is desirable, from the standpoint of ultimate stability of the corrected occlusion, that at the end of active treatment the lower incisor crowns are no nearer to the inner surface of the lower lip than at the commencement, indeed, were it not for considerations of general facial anaesthetics, it might be preferable that they should be slightly lingual of their original relationship to the lower lip.

It follows that, when closing space in Stage 2, the labial segments may need to be retracted far enough to compensate for the anticipated forward shift of the dental arches in Stage 3. The over-retraction must be accomplished without losing the edge-to-edge incisor, or the Class I buccal, relationship achieved in Stage 1.

Nevertheless, the Stage 3 reaction will not be the same in every case. The direction and degree of the required apical movements in Stage 3 and the root areas of the units involved differ from case to case, even within the Class II category. The differences increase when Class I and Class III malocclusions are met, or the balance of reciprocal apical anchorage for the multi-extraction case is assessed.

To these variables must be added the facts that the amount of space to be closed during Stage 2 can vary from case to case and that spacing is not always evenly distributed within each quadrant.

With so many variables involved it is inadvisable to recommend a standard way in which Stage 2 elastics should be applied. Inter- and intra-maxillary rubbers must be employed differentially, the various possible combinations being at the discretion of the operator, who works from his knowledge of anchorage and who must first clearly decide as to the precise nature of his intentions. It is possible only to provide some hints that might be of help in judging which elastics should be applied where.

The most typical situation to be found at the end of Stage 1 is that the incisor relationship is edge-to-edge, the buccal occlusion in either Class I or mild Class III relationship, with some fairly evenly distributed space in the extraction sites. The application of upper and lower *intra*-maxillary elastics only in this situation tends to have the greatest effect on the lower incisors which, having small root area, become more readily retracted than the upper incisors, thereby recreating an over-jet. The addition of *inter*-maxillary elastics each side reinforces the retraction of the upper incisors whilst, at the same time, giving added posterior support to the lower arch. The result is a balance of forces which maintains both the reduction of overbite and the established edge-to-edge incisor relationship.

The complex of rubbers built up by the inter- and intra-maxillary elastics, three each side, forms the shape of the letter Z (*Fig.* 4.1).

If this pattern is varied, the operator must be

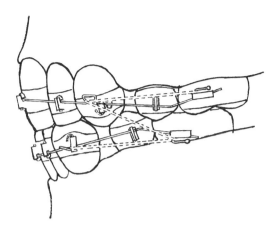

Fig. 4.1. General arrangement of the mechanics of Stage 2 of treatment. Archwires are of 0·018 in or 0·020 in gauge wire. The Z complex of space closing elastics is shown by broken line, since the pattern is subject to occasional variation (*see* text).

aware of all the consequences. It may be, or may seem to be, desirable that unilateral intra- or inter-maxillary elastics should be employed. It may be, or may seem to be, advisable to use a Class II inter-maxillary elastic one side and a Class III the other. These are, however, methods commonly employed to augment the correction of minor centre line discrepancies which are effective. It follows that where no centre line shift is present the use of unilateral rubbers may well create that fault.

The temptation to use unilateral rubbers, other than for centre line correction, is usually promoted by the spacing on one side becoming closed before the other. In these circumstances, precaution must be taken against unintentional dislocation of the centre lines by reinforcing anchorage in appropriate areas.

(i) Where unilateral space closure occurs in either dental arch, with no attendant centre line shift, a light intra-maxillary elastic could be kept on the closed side to counter the possibility of the archwire being pulled to the opposite side with an upset of arch symmetry, which might occur with the wearing of an intra-elastic on the open side only. If, however, the archwire on the closed side is held to the second bicuspid bracket by bypass clamp only whilst an intra-maxillary elastic is being worn, there exists the probability of overclosure of the space with some lingual displacement of the bicuspid.

(ii) It is desirable therefore, that the archwire pattern should be changed on the closed side so that the bracket of the second bicuspid can be fully engaged. The patterns of the archwire bends on the closed side become those later described for Stage 3 archwires, having a combined molar offset and height adjustment bend between molar and bicuspid and a further bend opposite the contact point between cuspid and bicuspid. On the open side the pattern remains as before, bypassing the bicuspid bracket slot. It must be seen that the anterior section of archwire, under this arrangement, does not slope to one side giving more depressive force to the incisors on one side than the other. On the closed side space must be prevented from reopening by distal turndown of the archwire, or ligation of lingual cleats by continuous ligature. With this archwire arrangement it is necessary to apply an intra-maxillary elastic on the open side only.

(iii) In order to reduce the effect of lateral drag by the unilateral elastic in the above circumstances, the anchorage value of the labial segment can be increased by fitting an uprighting spring to the cuspid on the side to which shift is anticipated. The spring should be designed to move the cuspid apex distally and, by reaction, the crown mesially, the latter action supporting the remainder of the labial segment.

(iv) Similar action to that of (iii) above, wherein uprighting springs are employed to give bodily control to units and provide a braking effect, can be taken in respect of the posterior segment on the side of closure. Additional anchorage support can be given to this segment against the possible effects of continued Class II mechanics by the placement of an uprighting spring on the second bicuspid on that side. This time the spring is designed to produce mesial apical movement and the leverage so supplied counters the pull of the Class II elastic (*Fig.* 4.2).

It is perhaps worth pointing out that, since the lateral incisors often require distal apical movement, advantage can be taken of this fact to further reinforce the anchorage value of the labial segment against displacement by a unilateral elastic pull. An uprighting spring can be fitted for this purpose, in addition to that on the cuspid, to prevent any swing towards the open side. The cuspid spring alone, however, will usually suffice for the purpose.

Methods of reinforcing the anchorage value of

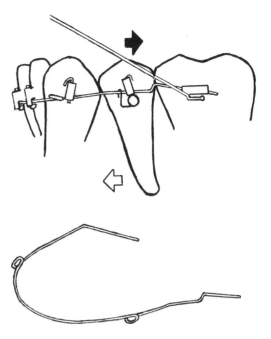

Fig. 4.2. Unilateral closure of space. On the open side, the anchor bend remains the Stage 1 or 2 pattern, bypassing the second bicuspid bracket. On the closed side, the bicuspid bracket slot is engaged, requiring a combined height adjustment and molar offset bend. The posterior anchor value on the closed side can be improved by the fitting of an uprighting spring for mesial root movement of the second bicuspid. Crown reaction from this auxiliary would be in the direction shown by the black arrow, root reaction by the white.

the whole of a labial segment against over-retraction when closing large amounts of residual space in the buccal regions will be discussed later where they most apply, namely, Class I treatments and the lower arch of Class III cases.

The use of uprighting springs in the capacity of brakes is a matter deserving considerable study when using the Begg appliance. In the mechanical field of orthodontics the direct action of components receives much attention, to a point where the orthodontist can become inclined to notice nothing else. The indirect or reciprocal actions often excite too superficial and hurried a study. Nowhere is it more important to work out to the full all action, particularly the reciprocal, than in the Stage 2 procedures of the Begg technique with its numerous variations on a theme.

During Stage 2 care must be taken, when the dental arches become shortened by the closure of space, that the anchor bends do not migrate too close to the mesial of the molar tubes, obstructing continuation of movement, or that the ends of the archwires do not produce the same effect, by impinging on the gingival tissues in the second molar region or upon the mesial aspect of the upper second molars.

Firm interproximal contacts should result from the Stage 2 space closure process. Over-closure of the extraction spaces should be avoided. Overtight contacts, or slipped contacts, will interfere with efficiency of root paralleling to be carried out during the next stage of treatment (Stage 3).

In order to avoid slipped contacts in cases of early unilateral space closure, archwires of 0·020 in or 0·018 in are preferred to 0·016 in. It will be recalled that, in the circumstances of unilateral closure, the archwire is seated fully into the bracket slot of the second bicuspid on the side of closure. If the smaller gauge of wire is used in association with continued Class II or intra-maxillary elastics, sufficient play is permitted within an 0·020 in bracket slot to allow mild overlap of cuspid and bicuspid to occur.

Centre Line Correction

Centre line discrepancies can be of major or minor proportions and confined to one dental arch or, where both arches contribute, can be in the same or opposite directions.

It must first be determined by reference to the estimated centre of the face whether the discrepancy is confined to one arch or due, in some measure, to both. If one arch only is involved, shifts of 2 mm and above can be regarded as major and may well need independent measures for correction, whilst those of 2 mm or under as minor and often self-correcting.

Where both centres are 1 mm out in opposite directions, although combining to produce a discrepancy of 2 mm, the amount in each arch is small and correctable without resorting to the separate movement of individual units.

Minor centre line discrepancies are often to be found in dental arches with good interproximal contacts on one side but slight lingual or buccal displacements of one or more units on the other, the teeth of the labial segment tilting towards the side of the malposed tooth or teeth. In these instances it will usually be found, following bicuspid extraction and general tooth alignment,

that more space exists on the side that was best aligned in the original condition than on the other. It can be anticipated that the application of the intra- and inter-maxillary elastics in Stage 2 will complete closure on the side to which the centre has shifted, before completion of closure on the side opposite. None of the methods mentioned earlier to *prevent* centre line movement should be used. The intra-maxillary rubber on the side which closes first can be discontinued, but inter-maxillary traction is continued bilaterally as before. In the lower arch the continuation of Class II mechanics brings forward the posterior teeth, which movement, through the existence of interproximal contacts on the side of closure, eventually induces a corrective swing of the centre line.

Minor shifts of the centre lines, such as discussed above, can also be inadvertantly introduced during the treatment process. In most cases they can be regarded as self-correcting, in that the standard Stage 2 procedures are usually sufficient to eliminate the fault. It should be realized, however, that the shift of the buccal teeth on the side of closure, together with the labial segment, will not occur quickly. If there is a foreseeable danger that the space on the open side will become closed before the desired shift has taken place, the movement of independant units of the labial segment may need to be undertaken.

In all instances of centre line correction there must be room not only to accommodate the labial segment in its corrected position, but also to allow for any allied movement of anchorage units that can be foreseen as stemming from the mechanics employed.

Where minor displacements of centre lines affect both arches Stage 2 is carried out, closing all residual space. Should the discrepancy still exist after this, the inter-maxillary elastic on one side is changed in its direction of pull from Class II to Class III, the other remaining Class II as before. This is the one situation where it is not imperative to have space available on the side to which a centre is to be moved.

A Class III inter-maxillary elastic, applied to the appropriate side, can also correct a minor centre line discrepancy which is confined to the upper arch only. In this instance all space should be closed on the side to which the centre has shifted whilst some space still exists on the opposing side. The Class III rubber will move the upper posteriors

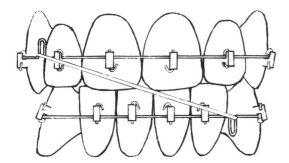

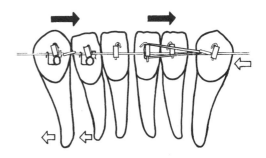

Fig. 4.3. Diagonal inter-maxillary elastic for the correction of the centre line of both arches. Centre line discrepancies of this kind have usually been promoted, either through the use of uncorrelated archwires, or inaccurately aligned buccal tubes, causing a lack of coordination between the anterior curvatures.

Fig. 4.4. Centre line correction by movement of individual or small group units. Following retraction by light intra-maxillary elastic of the left cuspid, the remaining units are moved by the combined action of uprighting springs and elastic ligature. The action must not be obstructed by the inter-maxillary hooks and the archwire must be firmly held at the distal of the molar tubes. The direct action is shown by the black arrows, the indirect by the white.

on that side mesially and, through interproximal contact, the teeth of the labial segment also.

When using intra- or inter-maxillary elastics, atypically or asymmetrically, for centre line correction, the operator must not become distracted by the need to eliminate the centre line fault, forgetting all else. The total action of any selected complex must be beneficial and not eliminate one fault at the expense of introducing another.

With this thought in mind, it may be helpful to assist the balance of anchorage by the addition of further auxiliaries. The action of the unilateral Class III elastic in the above example can be augmented by the fitting of an uprighting spring for distal movement of the upper cuspid root on the side to which the centre line is displaced, i.e. the same side as the Class III elastic. The lower cuspid on the same side can be supported against retraction by the placement of an uprighting spring, also for distal root movement. This action would prevent possible dislocation of the lower centre line. If the uprighting spring on the upper cuspid is to be allowed to produce some mesial movement of the crown of that tooth, there must be no obstruction from the inter-maxillary hook, which must be placed slightly to the mesial of the cuspid bracket.

There may be occasions when it is seen that, with the patient in occlusion, the upper and lower dental arches are swung in opposite directions a little, so that anteriorly the centres are not co-incident. This can come about through slight inaccuracy of molar tube alignment or failure to correlate archwires, but can be corrected readily

by the use of an anterior diagonal elastic worn between opposing upper and lower cuspid hooks in the appropriate direction for the desired correction (*Fig.* 4.3).

Major centre line shifts will not be corrected by the space closure procedures of Stage 2; the teeth of the offending segment or segments will need independent and individual movement, one or two teeth at a time. The mechanics for the process may well cause a temporary interruption of the general treatment progress, which can only be resumed after the centre line problem has been eliminated.

The cuspid, on the side to which the centre is to be moved, can be retracted with a very light pressure intra-maxillary elastic worn between molar hook and the tag of the cuspid lock pin. The light pressure and free tilting of the cuspid reduces serious risk of forward movement of the posterior anchor teeth.

Concurrent with the above movement the opposite cuspid is equipped with an uprighting auxiliary for distal movement of the apex which, reciprocally, drives the crown mesially.

Once the first cuspid has been retracted sufficiently it is tied back and the central and lateral incisors on the same side moved into contact by use of elastic thread between the tag of the central incisor lock pin and the inter-maxillary hook. Thereafter the remaining central and lateral can be assisted in the same manner and the same direction, if this should still be necessary (*Fig.* 4.4).

This method can be applied to either dental arch. It must be seen, however, that the intended movement is not obstructed by the inter-maxillary hooks and that neither of these has been tied to the archwire. Prevention of archwire swing to left or right through the buccal tubes must be accomplished, in this situation, by turning the distal ends round the posterior of the tubes.

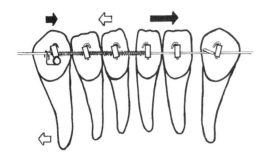

Fig. 4.5. An alternative system to that shown in *Fig.* 4.4, employing an active coil spring between the central incisors to move left central and lateral to the left, following independant retraction of the cuspid on that side. The uprighting spring on the right cuspid assists anchorage support. Closed coils between right central, lateral and cuspid prevent slipped contacts, but will eventually be made active following correction of the teeth on the left.

If there should be any doubt concerning the ability of the posterior teeth to stand up to the anchorage demands of centre line correction, the main archwire may be adapted to engage the second bicuspid brackets in the manner of a Stage 3 archwire. Further security can be added by placing uprighting springs, for mesial root movement, on the second bicuspids which can thereafter only move mesially under bodily control.

As a substitute for the rather cumbersome arrangement described above, some orthodontists have experimented successfully with small coil springs to carry out the same independent tooth movements in centre line correction in a manner similar to that used in other techniques (*Fig.* 4.5).

Major centre line corrections, therefore, may interrupt general progress and demand of the orthodontist some local improvization. His concern must be not only to correct the centre line but also to judge that the mechanics involved do not spoil other tooth relationships through the movement of anchorage units.

Stage 2 in Relation to Treatment of Class I and Class III Malocclusions

In the treatment of Class II malocclusions the tooth movements combined with anchorage responses are such as to ensure that, at the conclusion of Stage 1, there will be little excess space to close in Stage 2 in most instances.

Class I overcrowding cases may call for extraction, but there is no overjet to reduce and consequently there is less demand on available posterior anchorage. The result could be that there remain a high proportion of the original space created by extraction following general tooth alignment in mild discrepancy cases.

In such circumstances the arbitrary use of the Z-complex of inter- and intra-maxillary elastics would cause unnecessary retroclination of the labial segments. In order to avoid such 'dishing in' it is necessary to 'reverse anchorage' by making the anterior teeth more resistant to movement than the posteriors. This is done by applying lingual torque auxiliaries, either to the upper or lower labial segments, or both, which ensure against lingual or palatal tilting and promote greater anterior anchorage. These are the spurred arches, as used in the upper arch in Stage 3 and the lower torque arch shown in *Fig.* 4.7. Both can be applied almost passively to the anteriors, since they will automatically become active should any incisor retraction take place.

As an alternative, or addition, to the above arrangement, cuspid uprighting springs for distal root movement can be added. These will support the cuspids, and consequently the labial segments, against further retraction by Stage 2 space closing rubbers.

Lower cuspid support may become necessary once the lower labial segment has been so positioned as to compensate for any anticipated forward movement of the lower arch which may result from reaction to the mechanics of Stage 3. At this point the lower cuspids are usually distally inclined, in some occlusions more so than in others. The distal inclination may worsen, not through further retraction, but as a result of the continued anterior depressive force from the archwire against the slanting brackets, which can cause the cuspid apices to move further mesially. If excessive and unnecessary tilt is to be avoided, mildly active springs for distal root movement should be applied (*Fig.* 4.6).

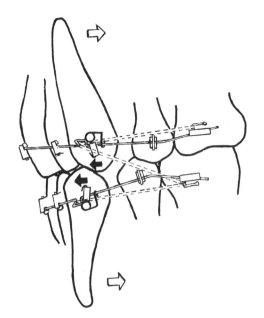

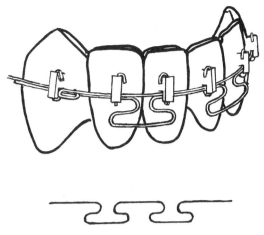

Fig. 4.7. An auxiliary for lingual root torque of lower incisors. Apart from active application, passive use can be made to prevent over-retraction of the lower labial segment.

Fig. 4.6. Use of distal root movement of cuspids to augment anterior anchorage so as to minimize risk of over-retraction of the labial segment by space closing elastics. Crown reaction is in the direction of the black arrows.

An anchorage problem related to the closure of large amounts of extraction space may also arise in the lower arch of some Class III conditions. The lower labial segment may have to support Class III elastic traction to correct reverse overjet and assist forward movement of the upper posterior teeth and, at the same time, support lower intra-maxillary elastics to close what may be a considerable amount of lower arch space. It could happen that the combined action of the four rubbers might threaten over-retraction of the lower labial segment, not so much by lingual crown movement but by continued transferrence of the root apices labially. To prevent this occurrence a lower lingual torque auxiliary is fitted (*Fig.* 4.7). The lower labial segment is then supported against further tilt from either set of elastics. In the lower arch the continued use of the intra-maxillary elastics will thereafter cause the posterior teeth to move forward rather than the anteriors to be retracted.

Chapter 5

Objectives and mechanics of the third phase of treatment (Stage 3)

The third stage of treatment should only be commenced after the objectives of the preceding stages, involving general alignment, correction of arch relationship and space closure, have been completed. The purpose of this last phase of active treatment is to promote, or restore, the axial inclination of those teeth that were, or have become, tilted.

The mechanics of Stage 3 are more complex than for the previous ones, involving the application of many auxiliaries (*Fig.* 5.1). Because of this fact, many orthodontists prefer to assemble the full apparatus in stages involving more than one visit. It is important that the entire assembly is secure and not, through hasty application or carelessness, liable to breakdown.

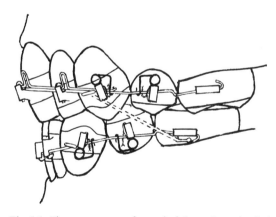

Fig. 5.1. The appearance of a typical Stage 3 mechanical composition, showing upper anterior palatal root torque auxiliary and paralleling springs in position. The tooth positions at this third stage can be compared to those in Stages 1 and 2, shown in *Figs.* 3.1 and 4.1.

The Fitting of Stage 3 Main Archwires

As soon as Stage 2 of treatment has been completed, the archwires are removed and replaced by Stage 3 archwires which differ in pattern and role to their predecessors. Stage 3 archwires are intended to fulfil a near passive role as stabilizers of the already obtained general alignment and vertical height adjustment. As such, they should be fully engaged in all brackets, including those of the second bicuspids, and will be made of 0·018 in or 0·020 in wire.

Because the archwires used in Stage 3 engage the second bicuspid brackets, there will need to be vertical compensation for the difference in height between the bicuspid bracket slot and the mesial of the anchor bend, due to the angle at which the anchor section of archwire emerges from the large molar tube. The adjustment is achieved by a bayonet bend which, at the same time, can be made to form a small molar offset in the opposite plane. The double effect is obtained by inserting the offset at 45° to the plane of the arch. The bends are placed midway between the mesial of the molar tube and the second bicuspid bracket. The pattern that emerges is that shown in the diagrams of the Stage 3 archwires (*Fig.* 5.2). If, however, the vertical positioning and relation to one another of the molar and bicuspid attachments is not as recommended, but is in some way unconventional (for example, if the molar tube has been placed exceptionally far to the gingival) the height adjustment arrangement will have to be altered to suit the circumstances.

The anchor bends are reduced at this stage, being only slightly active and acting more as an anti-tilt mechanism than as positive levers. The same section of wire is given slight toe-in, sufficient for anti-rotational control but not active, unless rotation of the molar is intended.

In order to maintain the anterior teeth in their edge-to-edge position, it is often necessary that the Stage 3 archwires carry, in addition to the posterior anchor bends, further bends of some 5° placed midway between cuspid and second bicuspid brackets. These bends carry the archwires towards the necks of the upper and lower anterior teeth, maintaining a light depression force on them. Unless this is done there will be a tendency for loss of overbite reduction. Should the edge-to-edge incisor relationship be lost in this way, it will be a time consuming concern to have to remove the Stage 3 multiple auxiliaries, adjust the main archwires and then reassemble the entire mechanism.

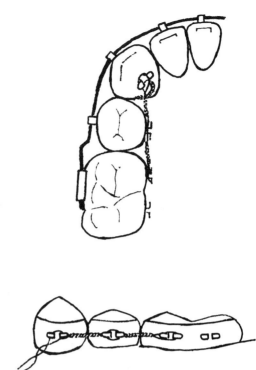

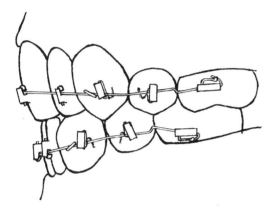

Fig. 5.2. The main archwires for Stage 3 in 0·020 in high tensile wire, with height adjustment bends mesial to the molars so as to seat the archwire passively in the bicuspid brackets. There is also a 5° bend in each archwire midway between the cuspid and bicuspid brackets either side to carry the anterior of the archwires gingivally as a precaution against possible loss of the edge-to-edge incisor relationship during Stage 3.

The Stage 3 archwires will be of ideal form, with correct anterior curvature and no expansion of the intercuspid width. They will be symmetrical with no expansion across the molar width, indeed the upper archwire may actually be contracted in this area by approximately 5 mm. The need for contraction will depend upon the presence of an upper anterior torquing auxiliary, since the contraction of the main archwire is to compensate for possible expansion stemming from that auxiliary. The amount of expansion derived will, in turn, depend upon the degree of activity placed in the spurs of the torquing arch.

The Stage 3 archwires will carry inter-maxillary traction hooks of the ring pattern, mesial to and in contact with the cuspid brackets, bent in the plane of the archwire.

The upper and lower Stage 3 archwires are fitted and firmly ligated into all brackets, using

Fig. 5.3. Continuous ligature tie applied to lingual cleats to prevent the reopening of the extraction sites in reaction to the root-paralleling springs.

0·009 in or 0·010 in soft ligature wire. The objective is to ensure, before auxiliaries are added, that the archwires fit snugly into the bracket slots. There should be no suggestion of partial bracket engagement. If necessary, the wires should be left in position for a week and at the end of that time the ligatures changed or tightened, until full bracket engagement has been achieved. Once this has been accomplished, the auxiliaries can be fitted.

It is necessary at this stage of the procedure to take steps to prevent the extraction spaces from reopening in response to the action of the root paralleling springs. Molars, bicuspids and cuspids can be ligated on the lingual or palatal side by a continuous ligature tied to the lingual cleats on each of the three teeth in all four quadrants (Fig. 5.3). Some orthodontists prefer an elastic chain to a steel ligature. If this is done it is important that there is little tension in the chain, because the teeth may then be brought into tight contact. If contacts become too tight the uprighting of the teeth, that is to follow, will be obstructed, since more space will be required in the dental arch for the upright teeth than the tilted.

Again, there are others who do not find either elastic chains or ligatures a necessity, preferring to turn the archwires gingivally round the posterior of the buccal tubes. If this is done, it must be realized that the buccal tube should not be used to help form the bend, since bending the archwire tightly round the tube will shorten the arch length and so promote an overclosure of the extraction spaces, producing the same stultification to uprighting as that described above. Allowance must be made for this and, assuming that the extraction spaces have been fully closed in the first place, the plier beaks must be used to initiate the bend. The pliers must be held at the appropriate angle, so that the archwire end is not turned to engage the buccal surface of the molar, yet not stand away so as to irritate or ulcerate the cheek. If the end of the archwire is brought into active contact with the molar the penalty will be unwanted root torque or rotation.

If there are any wrong band heights or placements this is the last occasion when correction can easily be carried out before the auxiliaries are fitted.

The Stage 3 auxiliaries will only be fitted when full bracket engagement has been gained on all teeth, even if this means waiting for a week or so until this object has been accomplished. Class II mechanics are continued during any pre-Stage 3 procedure such as that mentioned above. Until the auxiliaries are actually fitted the Class II elastic pressures can be kept down to 50 g, or even less, in order not to break the patient's routine and to assist in the maintainance of overbite reduction. There is no point in placing unnecessary strain on the lower arch anchorage during periods when there is neither overjet to reduce nor reciprocal action of auxiliaries to counterbalance.

Once full bracket engagement has been achieved on all teeth, the next phase of Stage 3 assembly can begin. This involves the addition of spring auxiliaries for the correction of the axial inclinations of teeth. Any of the teeth may require such correction, but those most commonly involved, as far as mesio–distal root movement is concerned, are the lateral incisors, cuspids and bicuspids of both dental arches. As for bucco–lingual root adjustment, the teeth most commonly involved are the upper central incisors and, to a lesser extent, the upper laterals.

The Fitting of Anterior Torquing Auxiliaries

It is reasonable, where anterior torquing auxiliaries are indicated, to fit them as the next phase of Stage 3 assembly. They lie parallel to the main archwires and both are pinned (with hook pins) or ligated together into the bracket channels. Some root paralleling springs will overlie both the main and auxiliary archwires and it is therefore logical to fit the latter first.

The Fitting of Root Paralleling Auxiliaries

Once any required anterior torque auxiliary has been fitted, the paralleling springs for mesio–distal root adjustment of the cuspids and bicuspids are

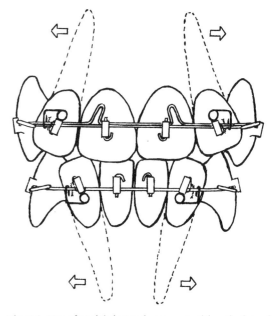

Fig. 5.4. Use of uprighting springs to reposition the lateral incisor apices. The roots of these teeth tend to be displaced mesially during overbite and overjet adjustment during the first two treatment stages.

added to the assembly. Usually at a slightly later date, the uprighting springs to correct the apical position of the upper and lower lateral incisors are fitted. These are usually required because the lateral incisor apices tend to move mesially and their crowns distally, as a reaction to the depression force applied to reduce overbite during the first two stages of treatment. The root apices of the upper laterals may be displaced towards the mid-line in the first instance, in which case the need to correct will be even more apparent. Correction will add to the stability of the incisors after discontinuation of retention (*Fig.* 5.4).

The movement of the lateral incisor apices can be left until last, because of their relatively small root area and consequent ease of correction.

Anterior Torquing Auxiliaries (Upper)

The pattern of the auxiliary will depend upon its purpose. Sometimes the central incisor apices are to be moved palatally, sometimes the lateral apices

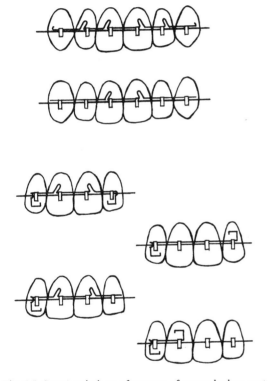

Fig. 5.5. Some variations of pattern of upper incisor root torque auxiliary to meet differing combinations of directional requirements.

require similar correction. At other times, the central apices are to be moved palatally, whilst those of the laterals are to be moved labially and this may be a bilateral or unilateral concern. The permutations of possibility in the pattern of the torquing agent are best shown by graphic illustration, which makes their individual purpose, technical construction and fitting almost self-evident (*Figs.* 5.5 and 5.6).

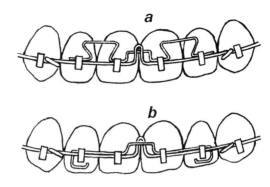

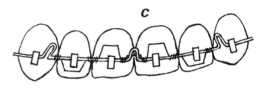

Fig. 5.6. Some examples of alternative mechanics for incisor torque, showing the use of a midline spur in the main archwire, against which to promote activity of an auxiliary or wound-on spring.

Supplementary to the graphic illustrations, it is necessary to describe in detail the construction and fitting of a typical example. That chosen for the purpose is the auxiliary for the palatal movement all four upper incisors.

The wire employed is 0·016 in high tensile steel. Some prefer to use 0·014 in wire in the interests of light pressure application. The larger gauge is, however, recommended because the resulting auxiliary is more stable to handle, being less liable to loss of shape or activity.

Vertical spurs are bent into the wire to conform with points just distal to the central and lateral incisor brackets. These spurs will transmit the torque forces, but do not generate them and need to be no more than 3 to 4 mm in height. The movement force is derived from the twist, or torque, generated in the horizontal sections of the auxiliary archwire when the spurs are applied to the labial surfaces of the incisors. The point about which the teeth pivot is determined by the position of the bracket slots, which hold both the auxiliary and the main archwire.

In order that torque be set up, the spurs must be at an angle to the labial surfaces of the incisors, which means in turn that they will be angled to the plane of the horizontal sections of the auxiliary. The angle made between the spurs and the plane

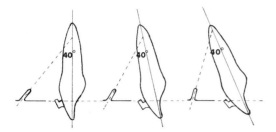

Fig. 5.7. Diagram to show the angle made to the long axis of an upper central incisor by the spur of a palatal root-torque auxiliary. By maintaining the angle at 40°, the initial force application is kept constant from case to case, although the spur angle to the horizontal plane decreases the more the tooth is retroclined. An arbitrary standard angle between spur and the archwire plane, results in pressure application varying from individual to individual.

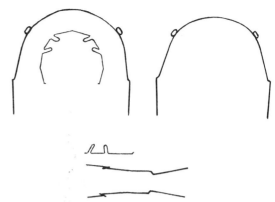

Fig. 5.8. The pattern of Stage 3 archwires, viewed from the occlusal and laterally; also a four spur torque auxiliary which is kept contracted relative to the curvature of the main arch.

of the archwire should not be determined by universal standard regardless of the degree of retroclination of the upper incisors. A standard can be applied so long as it is related to the individual patient. If the spurs are placed at 40° to the long axis of the incisors a reasonable pressure is exerted from the points of view of both the rate of apical movement and the strain on anchorage. Keeping the angle of the spurs to the long axes of the teeth as a constant will mean, since tooth angulation varies, that they will subtend varied angles to the archwire horizontal in different cases, but apply the same initial force in all cases (*Fig.* 5.7).

If more enthusiastic pressures are employed the result will be a tendency to greater expansion and buccal roll of the auxiliary archwire in the buccal regions, where the reciprocal effects will be felt. Even with the more modest pressures some expansionary reaction is to be expected, in consequence of which the auxiliary is kept contracted (*Fig.* 5.8). It will be recalled that the main archwire may also need to be kept contracted across the molar region as a further compensation for the expansion created by the anterior torque auxiliary. It is doubtful whether contraction of both the main archwire and the auxiliary will be required if pressure application is modest. The orthodontist himself will come judge the compensation needed in his case. He may well find that contraction of an 0·016 in auxiliary is sufficient and that the main archwire can be kept passive in the buccal tubes.

The expansion and rolling effects from active anterior torque spurs was far more significant in the days when the spurs were bent into the main archwire rather than an auxiliary. In addition to the spurs being placed at an angle to the labial surfaces of the incisors, they are also angled towards the centre of the labial surfaces in order to minimize any unwanted rotatory effect. Once the anterior torque auxiliary has been formed it is fitted into the incisor and cuspid brackets above the main archwire.

The upper central incisors are pinned with third stage lock pins (hook pins), or ligated first, with the ends of the auxiliary protruding from the mouth. The whole auxiliary is then turned over and spread to engage the cuspid brackets. The free ends of such an active and contracted sectional arch will need to be controlled to prevent impingement and damage to the gingivae. This control can be provided by nurse or patient on the one side, whilst the other is ligated into the cuspid bracket slot.

The ends of the auxiliary should terminate 2 to 3 mm distal to the cuspid brackets. These ends may need to be turned slightly inwards so that there is no sharpness or roughness that might irritate the buccal mucosa. Any such turn, or terminal loop, should not be allowed to interfere with the action of the uprighting springs to cuspids or bicuspids, which have yet to be fitted.

In the case of an upper torquing auxiliary whose action is confined to palatal root movement of the central incisors only, the free ends usually terminate distal to the cuspid brackets, in the manner described above, if the most positive reaction is to be obtained. Termination distal to the lateral brackets is less assured, but may not be entirely ineffective in cases with pronounced anterior arch curvature.

It should be mentioned that the spurs need not necessarily be on the distal side of the incisor brackets. It may be helpful after incisors have been previously rotated to place spurs on that side of the bracket which discourages relapse and this might mean the mesial rather than the distal.

It must be realized that the action of the spurs will be not only to move the incisor apices palatally, but also the crowns of those teeth towards the labial, unless the latter movement is actively prevented. The upper dental arch will supply some of the anchorage required, but this will probably be inadequate and the continuation of Class II mechanics is necessary.

If labial root torque is applied to any of the incisors it will help counterbalance the effects on anchorage of palatal root torque directed to other incisors of the same segment.

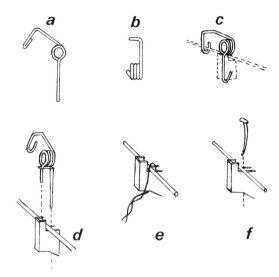

Fig. 5.9. *a, b* and *c,* The root paralleling spring. *d,* The combination lock pin and spring. *e,* The application of 0·010 in soft wire ligature to secure archwire to bracket, prior to placement of uprighting spring. *f,* The lingual lock pin, designed as an alternative to a ligature for securing the archwire.

Uprighting or Root Paralleling Springs

These springs are made from 0·014 in or 0·012 in hard SS (stainless steel) wire and, for accuracy of finish, are preferably machine rather than hand wound (*Figs.* 5.9 *a,b* and *c*).

The 0·012 in springs are reserved for the uprighting of teeth of small root area, for example lower incisors. They have the advantage, for the anterior regions, of being slightly less bulky than springs of 0·014 in gauge. The choice of which gauge spring to use and where, is largely a matter of personal attitude and conviction and, so long as force application is kept within reason, is unlikely to affect the outcome of treatment.

The springs of either gauge are prefabricated with three full coils wound on a core of 1 mm wire. The diameter of the coils is significant in that, if too large, they will interfere to a greater extent with the gingival tissues when in position in the brackets. The coils are wound, some in one direction and some in the other, so that whether the tooth to be uprighted is left or right, upper or lower, and whichever direction the root is to be moved, there is a spring form available which is appropriate.

The spring selected for a given tooth should be suited to the direction of root movement required and the direction of coil winding should be such that, when the spring is placed in the bracket slot,

the coils overlie the main archwire in the same manner as does the head of a lock pin. The arrangement acts as a secondary defence against the archwire escaping from the bracket slot. The primary defence is provided by the main archwire being tied into the bracket slot by 0·009 in or 0·010 in ligature. It is of great importance that the tooth be held securely onto the archwire, because the action of the uprighting spring will elevate the tooth above the general occlusal level, unless prevented. The coils of the spring alone are insufficient guarantee that the tooth will be properly held.

The ligature tags should be turned to lie beneath the archwire and care taken that they do not provide interference to the process of uprighting.

After selecting a spring with coils wound in the appropriate direction to overlap the archwire and suited to the direction of root movement required, the plain end is passed into the pin channel of the bracket. The other end carries an offset hook which is to be latched to the archwire. Before latching, the short lever arm carrying the hook should be set at an angle of 45° to the main archwire. This will give a reasonable force. For consistency in force application, spring deflection is measured against the plane of the archwire, not against the long axis angle of the tooth.

When the hook end is latched to the main archwire the short lever arm should lie parallel with the archwire. No part of the lever arm or coil should be imbedded in the gingival tissues, nor should there be any possibility that it might occur by pressure contact.

The end of the spring which has been placed in the pin channel of the bracket may be cut to the length of that channel, since once the other end has been hooked onto the archwire, the spring force set up will keep the spring in place. It is, however, probably better policy to leave enough wire at the bracket end of the spring to enable it to be turned round the bracket in the manner of a locking pin. Unless this is done, any spring which becomes accidentally unlatched will be lost, with attendant possible consequences. The active arm should be latched to the main archwire before turning the other end round the bracket. This avoids the introduction of unintentional rotation of the tooth.

The areas where the springs are fitted must be carefully examined to see that there are no projecting sharp ends.

The ready availability of machined prefabricated springs of uniform dimensions fortunately makes the inconsistencies of hand woven products a thing of the past. The shortening of the lever arm is a development which has done much to overcome accidental unlatching. This shortness, however, can be overdone and make the initial application of the auxiliary difficult.

As the action of the spring takes effect and the tooth becomes more upright, the latched end will move slightly along the archwire. Where adjacent teeth are to be uprighted in opposite directions, the latching arms will be hooked over the same inter-bracket span of the main archwire. As the teeth upright, the latching ends will move towards each other. They must not be allowed to come into contact, nor become obstructed by any other archwire bend, stop, offset or loop. In order to prevent contact, the spring ends should be at least 2−3 mm apart at the outset of movement.

Uprighting or root paralleling springs are available made with a combined locking pin (*Fig. 5.9d*). Displacement of the spring is prevented by turning the pin tag round the bracket instead of the end of the spring. There is also the lingual lock pin, designed to replace the ligature for retaining the main archwire when the spring auxiliaries are in use (*Fig. 5.9 f*). Both are a logical attempt to improve the assembly, but it is open to question whether any real improvement, from either the operative or the mechanical standpoint, has been brought about. The first arrangement, previously described, still seems the more secure and mechanically efficient.

Combined or compound uprighting springs have the disadvantage that the activity of one spring cannot be increased or decreased without altering that of the other.

The action sought from all these spring auxiliaries is to upright or parallel the roots of the teeth, but their reciprocal effect on the crowns must be taken into account. The crown end will be the first to respond, unless restrained, and will move in the opposite direction to that intended for the root. In the case of cuspids and second bicuspids, for example, whose roots are to be moved towards each other, the crowns will move apart, reopening the first bicuspid extraction sites, unless either the arch length is held by ligature to lingual buttons or cleats or the archwire is turned round the posterior of the buccal tubes on the molars.

The leverage applied to the roots can effect a shift of the whole of the dental arch. The combined action of palatal root torque to the upper incisors and distal movement of the apices of any of the buccal teeth is to cause arches to move anteriorly. It is because of this reaction, that both dental arches must be aligned and orientated to one another, to the lingual of their intended ultimate position, during Stages 1 and 2, thus allowing for the expected Stage 3 anchorage shift.

If some teeth, on the other hand, happen to require movement of their apices in a mesial or labial direction, the effect on anchorage of the auxiliaries employed will be to help counterbalance the effect of those for the opposite purpose.

It is often the case, therefore, that some of the uprighting forces happen to balance one another, thereby assisting anchorage problems; but this depends on circumstances and is not necessarily so. The total effect on anchorage of the third stage auxiliaries must be carefully assessed early in treatment planning.

It follows from considerations of anchorage that there can be a lateral loss of anchorage and that such matters are not confined to the antero–posterior dimension.

The possible use of unilateral uprighting springs

is a matter for cautious forethought, since the threat to the dislocation of the centre lines of the arches becomes very real under these circumstances.

The importance of uprighting springs in a braking role should be realized. Should one cuspid in one arch require distal apical movement, but not the cuspid of the opposite side, an uprighting spring should nevertheless be fitted to the latter which is only slightly active. This spring will become more active, and consequently resistant, if pressure develops through mesial crown movement on the active side, so aiding the main archwire and intermaxillary hooks in the preservation of the centre line position.

It will usually be safe policy to fit springs in matching pairs, unless a deliberate shift of a centre line is intended.

In this context, the value as braking agents of springs for the mesial movement of the second bicuspids of a first bicuspid extraction case is sometimes lost to sight. Even if these teeth do not require root movement, or if it has been completed, the presence of springs for mesial apical movement will help stabilize anchorage by becoming increasingly active should the arches be drawn anteriorly by other forces, providing resistance through bodily control.

Because of these considerations, it becomes almost conventional to place uprighting springs in Stage 3 on all but the central incisors and molars, as a minimal requirement.

Anterior Torquing Auxiliaries (Lower)

Auxiliary for Lingual Root Torque of Lower Incisors

One reaction to the depression force from the lower main archwire to the lower anteriors is to cause the apices of the lower incisors to move lingually. In consequence it is seldom required that this particular movement be actively produced by separate auxiliary.

The lower lingual root torque auxiliary, therefore, is more often employed to reinforce the anchorage value of the lower incisors against over-retraction, or to prevent undue displacement of their apices towards the labial, when active retraction agents are applied to the lower labial segment.

The need for increased anterior anchorage is most likely to arise in Class I or Class III treatments where extraction has provided space considerably in excess of that needed for general tooth alignment and where the claim on posterior anchorage is minimal.

The pattern of the auxiliary is shown in *Fig. 4.3*. It is constructed from 0·014 in or 0·016 in hard SS wire. The double spurs are suitably angled to the plane of the auxiliary to produce the required force value and the whole is kept contracted across the cuspid width. In short, the auxiliary is a slight modification, to suit the lower incisor region, of the upper palatal root torquing spurred arch.

In the treatment of Class I occlusions the provision of spurs to the upper or lower incisors prevent them from tilting should they threaten to become excessively retroclined (dished in) under the influence of inter- or intra-maxillary space closing forces. The presence of the spurs on the anterior teeth compels bodily retraction of the incisors, increasing their anchorage value relative to the posteriors, resulting in the closure of the extraction spaces more by the mesial movement of the latter than by the lingual shift of the former.

The above mechanical arrangement implies a reversal of the usual anchorage situation whereby the posterior teeth give the most resistance through provision of bodily control whilst the anteriors are allowed to tilt freely.

The treatment of Class III occlusions may also provide problems of excess space, particularly where first bicuspids have had to be removed from the lower arch. It can come about that lower intramaxillary rubbers need to be used concurrent with Class III elastics. The lower labial segment will be in receipt of the reciprocal forces of the combination. The crowns of the lower incisors and cuspids cannot retract indefinitely within the confines of their supporting bone, but the continued use of the elastics may cause their apices to progress further labially so that excessive retroclination comes about through root movement rather than crown. The lingual root torque auxiliary should be fitted if this occurrence is threatened.

Auxiliaries for Labial Root Torque of Lower Incisors

A common form of auxiliary for the labial root torque of lower incisors is shown in *Fig. 5.10*. It is constructed from 0·014 in hard SS wire and derives its force to the lower incisor tips by means

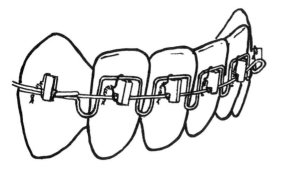

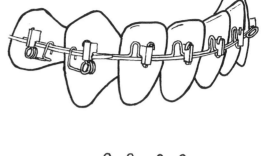

Fig. 5.11. An alternative auxiliary for labial root torque of lower incisors, which can be used for similar purposes as that shown in *Fig.* 5.10 and for correction of bucco—lingual apical displacement.

Fig. 5.10. Auxiliary for labial root torque of lower incisors. Apart from active application, the auxiliary can be used in an initially passive state to supplement anchorage against forces tending to displace the lower incisors labially.

of the interstitial loops sprung against the inner aspect of the main lower archwire.

The loops should be made so that they extend positively gingival to the main archwire to ensure continuous contact, but should not be extravagantly deep. If the loops are too large in the vertical dimension they will be liable to impinge on the gingivae. This can be circumvented by bending the ends of each loop away from the gingival tissues, but there still remains the problem of continued oral hygiene since extensive loops prevent the toothbrush from maintaining the tone of the soft tissues.

Lower incisors are usually labially inclined to various degrees. If, therefore, the vertical loops are bent at right angles to the horizontal, or fitting, sections of the auxiliary, it will be found to be active once ligated into position. If additional activity is needed, this can be very simply done. Using the fingers and thumbs of two hands, the loops are slightly parted from each other. This will have the effect of altering the angle of the loops to the fitting plane of the auxiliary.

As with other anterior root torque auxiliaries, it is probably wise to contract across the intercuspid width by generally increasing the curvature of the auxiliary, whilst maintaining the symmetry.

A second design of auxiliary for the same purpose is shown in *Fig.* 5.11. This is also constructed of 0·014 in hard SS wire. It would not

be wrong to use 0·016 in wire for either of these auxiliaries, but the smaller gauge is adequate for the movement of lower incisor roots with their small surface area.

In the case of this second pattern, the auxiliary accompanies the main archwire within the bracket slot, which must be deep enough to contain both. In order to avoid the introduction of minor rotations from the pressure of the spurs, the main archwire should be of 0·020 in gauge, which precisely fills the bracket slot. Using this gauge for the main arch will mean that there will be little space within the slot, in the vertical dimension, for the larger gauge of auxiliary.

The small size of the lower incisors leaves no latitude for error in the positioning of the vertical spurs, which must be placed as near the brackets as possible. Once again, posterior expansion is avoided by making the auxiliary to a somewhat smaller arc than that of the main archwire.

Symmetry of both the main archwire and the auxiliary is important, if the lower incisor apices and crowns are each to finish on the proper curve.

Broadly, there are three purposes for which either of these two auxiliaries might be fitted:

(1) As active agents to move the lower incisor roots labially and align their apices;

(2) As a means of reinforcing lower arch anchorage against forces which tend to displace that arch in a labial direction. The fitting of the auxiliary, even if almost passive, ensures that the lower labial segment cannot tilt labially. There will be bodily control of the lower incisors in this

direction. The more the lower labial segment tries to tilt labially under displacing forces, the more active the auxiliary becomes; and

(3) To assist in overbite reduction (*see* Chapter 8).

If the above are the theoretical reasons for which one or other of the lower labial root torque auxiliaries might be fitted, the next logical observation is to state under what circumstances the fitting becomes a practical necessity.

This is one of many similar issues which is under current debate. Unfortunately it is not uncommon 'for orthodontists to hold strong individual opinions as to the proper course of action in any given circumstance, yet to be at considerable variance with each other on the same issues.

As far as the use of the auxiliary for active labial root torque is concerned it has been previously stated that, during treatment Stages 1 and 2, the lower incisor roots move lingually, increasing their long axis angle to the mandibular plane. It would seem reasonable, therefore, that this displacement should be corrected. However, once bands have been removed and the teeth allowed to settle, the lower incisors erupt to reestablish overbite. This movement is accompanied by a readjustment of the lower incisor apical position towards the labial in all cases, other than perhaps Class III occlusions. It would seem pointless, therefore, to carry out by auxiliary a movement that nature will perform unaided, unless some further purpose is to be accomplished. One such purpose would be to bring into line the lower incisor apices, should they happen to be in disarray. A second purpose would be to bolster lower arch anchorage through deliberate labial root torque to the lower incisors. The two services can, of course, be rendered by the same auxiliary simultaneously. If neither of these actions is required, the lower incisor apices being already well aligned and lower labial segment so positioned at the commencement of Stage 3 that no real threat exists from subsequent lower arch anchorage loss, then no auxiliary need be fitted.

Correction of Mesial Tilt and/or Lingual Roll of Molars

The lingual roll of molars is a problem attending round arch banded appliances and is caused by forces which tend to elevate the buccal aspect of the molars. In the case of the Begg appliance, these forces develop through the anchor bends and inter-maxillary elastics and affect the lower arch more than the upper.

The degree of roll will depend upon the amount and duration of the applied forces, the original bucco—lingual root angle, the size of the root area and the amount of space afforded to the roots by the cross-sectional area of the bone in the molar region.

Most of these factors are to be seen at their most adverse in the second molar region. Here the original molar position is often one of marked lingual inclination before tooth movement is begun. There is ample space for the roots to be transferred further to the buccal and, as a rule, these second molars will need to be moved mesially two-thirds of the width of the first molar extraction spaces before the latter become closed.

The fact that archwires are kept expanded throughout the first and second stages of treatment, emanates from a desire to improve posterior anchorage whilst minimizing molar rolling. The amount of expansion given is insufficient to cause any widening of the dental arches, but enough to counter the lingual movement that would otherwise take place. The inter-maxillary elastics can be applied to a lingual hook or button on the molar band in order to produce another means of minimizing lingual roll. The round buccal tubes can be changed for ones of oval cross-section which accept an archwire doubled back on itself so that two lengths of archwire pass through the same tube. Although not entirely ineffective, this anti-roll mechanism is often bedevilled by lack of space in the vertical dimension in the lower second molar region and by the comparative instability of the double arch section. Molar rolling, tilting or rotation can therefore occur even though precautions have been taken to minimize it.

The archwire shown in *Fig.* 3.9 can be used for the correction of the faults, but, because of the coincidental introduction of frictional hazards, may have to perform its functions as a separate stage in treatment. The archwire takes the form of a recurved wire which bypasses the gingival side of the buccal tubes, curving back to enter the tubes from the posterior. If the recurved loops are angled buccally to the plane of the archwire, a combination of forces being set up once the archwire is in the tubes. The main archwire, passing gingival to the tubes, bears lingually on the molars. The section passing into the tubes is active towards the buccal. A torque force corrective of lingual roll is thereby imparted to the molars.

The same recurved section can be angled to assist correction of mesial molar tilt or mesio–lingual rotation. A helicle is often incorporated into the recurve bend, but would appear to contribute more to bulk than efficiency.

Chapter 6

Cephalometric interpretation of tooth movement

The study of radiographs, particularly from the lateral headplate, can provide valuable information for the orthodontist before, after and during treatment of the patient.

At the treatment planning stage, the lateral radiograph can assist in the detection of any potential limitations to the ideal positioning of the teeth which might arise from either the morphology or the relationship of the surrounding bony structures. Following treatment, the extent and relative success of the tooth movements accomplished can be demonstrated and the associated growth contribution assessed.

A major importance of the lateral skull radiograph is the guidance it can provide to the orthodontist during the actual progress of treatment. Clinical judgement can be enhanced through periodic monitoring of tooth positions with the aim of obtaining, at the conclusion of active treatment, the best possible natural stability of the dentition.

General Observations on the Stability of the Treated Occlusion

Before outlining examples of methods that can be used to derive information from lateral skull radiographs, some general observations are now given on those factors currently thought to influence the natural stability of the occlusion.

The object of orthodontic treatment, using the Begg or any other form of appliance, is not merely to straighten the individual teeth but to ensure that, in so doing, the dental arches as a whole are placed in such a relationship with their supporting and surrounding structures that the maximum chance of natural stability is given to the teeth in their new positions.

Any form of retainer appliance may be used to support the treated occlusion during the period of settling and tissue repair which follows the removal of the active appliance. Even the longest of retention periods, however, is no guarantee of continued permanent stability once the retainer has been discarded.

Since natural stability of the occlusion is preferable to indefinite artificial support by appliance, treatment must be planned and carried out with proper respect to all known factors governing that stability.

The lower labial segment provides the best key to the stable antero–posterior relationship of the dental arches in the facial skeleton, both before and after treatment. It is wise general treatment policy not to allow or promote the movement of this segment labially through arch expansion or anchorage failure. The relationship of the lower labial segment to the facial structures should be the same after treatment as before in the majority of cases. It might even be true to say that it should be slightly lingual to the original position. Lingual movement of 2–3 mm of the lower incisor crowns, where applicable to the case, does not lead to instability. Where alignment of the lower incisors is required, correction should be by mesio–distal, not labial, movement of these teeth.

When the lower incisors have been aligned and positioned to conform with the above concept, the remaining teeth of the lower arch and those of the upper are brought to coordinate with the lower incisors in their selected location. This may at times prove difficult in practice, and some may regard the rule as over-restricting. Genuine exceptions do exist, and it is tempting to make use of this fact to abandon the rule when it could and should be applied. Again, there is no doubt that what is good for the stability of the teeth after treatment is not necessarily also beneficial to general facial aesthetics.

Both the existence of the exceptions and the

consideration of facial aesthetics have led to the introduction of a modified ruling in respect of the post-treatment position of the lower labial segment. An allowance of plus or minus so many millimetres from the original lower central incisor tip position, as measured antero–posteriorly against a selected vertical plane or line, is permitted. Such a ruling certainly relieves the restrictions on the orthodontist, but he must take care that he uses the latitude, thus 'scientifically' granted, in the right context.

When lower incisors erupt they take up positions dictated by local environmental factors as they pertain at that particular time. General growth and local factors may alter the balance of that original environment and the teeth may react accordingly, but more often either the environment changes too little to encourage accompanying tooth movement, or one form or another of obstruction prevents the teeth from responding and perpetuates, partly or wholly, the existing situation.

It will be seen from Chapter 11 that the erupting lower incisors, once under the influence of the oral soft tissues, become rapidly and markedly more labially inclined than when contained within bone.

This natural tilt can be obstructed in a number of ways, one of which is that, particularly in cases of low anterior facial height, the tips of the lower incisors contact the palatal mucosa. Their full forward swing is impeded and they are likely to remain in that position, even when the facial height increases.

If subsequent growth in that dimension is adequate, the orthodontist will be able to take advantage of it and, having reduced overbite, to complete by appliance the full labial tilt of the lower incisors without penalty of subsequent relapse. He would, in this instance, be placing those teeth in a position antero–posteriorly that they would have occupied naturally, had the balance of their surroundings been favourable at the time of eruption.

The above situation, however, is the exception not the rule. In the majority of cases, the lower incisors are unobstructed during eruption and take up a position of balance which is correct and should not be subsequently altered. If alteration is carried out, involving movement of the lower incisor crowns labially in the interests, for example, of facial aesthetics, a measure of imbrication can be expected to develop in the long run. It is

possible that a bodily forward movement may be more stable than one involving only tilt.

Unfortunately, late imbrication of lower incisors can take place after apparently immaculate treatment procedures and even when space has been created by extraction. A mesial migration of teeth occurs as a natural process, designed perhaps to compensate for attrition which no longer takes place with modern diet. The amount of eventual imbrication may well be influenced by the type of accompanying mandibular growth taking place, the 'opening' form of growth rotation being more favourable than the 'closing', but unfortunately neither can be permanently promoted or changed by orthodontic treatment.

Through exceptions and uncertainties, the orthodontist is provided with an excuse, if he should be looking for one, for not worrying too much about the treated position of the lower anterior teeth antero–posteriorly.

It is surely desirable not to invite certain relapse when known measures can be taken to avoid or minimize the effect. Orthodontic treatment would indeed be easy if all that was called for was the arbitrary alignment of the teeth with no governing restrictions.

Close observation should be kept, therefore, at every stage of treatment with regard to the position of the lower anteriors and, at the same time, a watch maintained against unintentional expansion of the buccal teeth.

The lateral dimension of the dental arches should be checked by caliper measurements taken routinely across the inter-molar and inter-cuspid widths. A general shift of the lower arch labially is less easy to assess by direct measurement; indeed the use of clinical judgement alone may prove insufficiently reliable to determine whether or not the labial surfaces of the lower incisors have been brought nearer to the lower lip. This is particularly true where round archwires have been employed.

The depression force supplied through a round archwire to the lower incisors, which are usually labially inclined prior to treatment, causes the angle made between the long axes of these teeth and the mandibular plane to increase. This can be due, wholly or in part, to the lingual movement of their apices, but it is essential to know whether labial movement of their crowns has contributed, and if so by how much. It is here the clinical eye may be deceived, unless some supporting method of assessment is introduced.

The possession of lateral skull radiographs and tracings can be of considerable assistance in supplying the required information in these circumstances. Comparison can be made between the lateral headplate radiograph taken before tooth movement was started and any such subsequent radiograph obtained as treatment proceeds.

The first important point of assessment occurs towards the end of Stage 1, but before the extraction sites have been closed. It is of vital consequence that, should it be found that the crowns of the lower incisors have been advanced towards the lip, space still exists in sufficient quantity for their retraction to their proper location. In the case of the Begg technique the typical anchorage demands made by the mechanics of Stage 3 are such that by the conclusion of Stage 2 the incisors of the lower labial segment must be retracted well to the lingual of their final intended position with the upper incisors in an edge-to-edge relationship with them.

Further checks can be made in the same way at later stages, particularly as the final stage of treatment nears completion.

Use of Lateral Skull Radiographs and Tracings for Establishing the Antero–posterior Relationship of the Dentition to the Facial Skeleton

One renowned but unfortunate quality inherent in tracings of lateral skull radiographs is their inaccuracy. Lateral skull tracings can be inaccurate or very inaccurate, depending upon the methods employed in their production. This does not mean that no guidance of any value can ever be obtained through study and measurement of lateral radiographs. If appropriate measures are taken to ensure maximum potential accuracy, great support and confirmation can be given to clinical judgement. The inaccuracy referred to implies that the lateral skull radiograph and tracing cannot be regarded as constituting collectively a precision instrument. The orthodontist cannot therefore declare, on the grounds of cephalometric measurement, that he has moved the tips of the lower incisors in a given case, say 2·3753 mm to the labial. This would be taking the claim to four places of absurdity. He has, however, to plus or minus a millimetre, a useful indication of the effect of his treatment.

In order to ensure a proper degree of accuracy in interpreting tooth movement cephalometrically,

more than one set of reference points should be used and, if possible, more than one method of assessment, so that the object can be viewed in different ways and from several angles.

When the object of study is tooth movement, the truest interpretation results if the assumption is made, over the relatively short duration of active treatment, that no change in angular relationship occurs between planes of reference, due to growth or other causes. It can also be assumed that teeth do not change shape or alter their root-to-crown angle as a result of treatment. The outlines of, for example the incisors, can be transferred from one tracing in a series to the next and the reference points at the tip of crown and apex, which determine measurement of the long axis, correlated from tracing to tracing. Even if a mistake is made in interpreting root form, at least consistency is gained by repeating the mistake in exactly the same measure in subsequent tracings. This consistency does not necessarily attend uncorrelated tracings even when care has been taken to trace what appears to be there.

The number of reference points for lateral skull X-rays, recommended for use by orthodontists the world over, gives the strong impression that the introduction of yet another landmark is the result of some compulsive international conspiracy. Reputations have been enhanced by the selection of anatomical reference points which others have not heard of or have forgotten. Unhappily such points are often those which can only be found occasionally and with some uncertainty, even on the best quality radiograph.

Points used for reference must be those most easily identified with the greatest consistency from radiograph to radiograph, patient to patient and tracer to tracer.

Lines and Angles of Reference

Only three methods of detecting change, during or after treatment, are to be described in the following notes:

(1) The use of the APo line;
(2) The use of the NB line; and
(3) The use of the angle SNI.

All three can be used in association with the conventional lateral skull tracing, but can also supply useful immediate information at the chairside by the direct application to the radiograph of a ruler or protractor (*Fig. 6.1*).

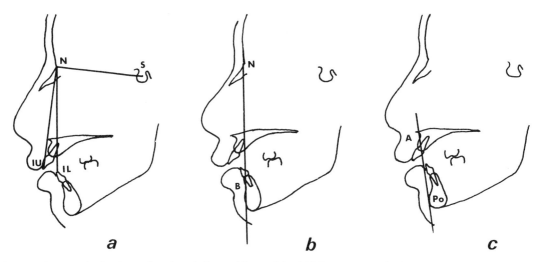

Fig. 6.1. Three methods of assessing the relative positions of the labial segments and subsequent alteration of position resulting from treatment. *a*, The angles SNI upper or lower. *b*, The NB line. *c*, The APo line (*for usage, see text*).

The APo Line

This line, drawn on a lateral skull tracing, connects point A with Pogonion and provides a reference against which either lingual or labial movement of the lower incisors crowns can be measured.

In the majority of cases, at the conclusion of treatment, the labial surfaces or incisal tips of the lower incisors should not occupy a position labial to their original relationship to the APo line. This would represent a strict adherence to the rules; there are many who advocate a latitude for the position of the lower central incisor tip after treatment of −3 to +2 mm relative to the APo line.

Much depends on how this latitude in interpreted. If the lower labial segment is moved a total of 2 to 3 mm labially during treatment, it is possible that with the closure of lower band spaces, together with the reestablishment of an overbite, that the degree of error would be accommodated.

On the other hand, over-free interpretation of the above latitude must increase the chance of lower incisor relapse and imbrication. For example, if the lower anteriors are initially found at −3 mm to the APo line and are moved to a new position at +3 mm, a total labial movement of 6 mm, the chances of permanent natural stability would seem to be very small.

In both the above examples the factors of mesial tooth migration and mandibular growth would also be adding their effect, for better or worse. At worst there could be the probability of late lower incisor imbrication, even where the rules had been strictly applied; at best there would be the chance that this detrimental effect might be avoided even if some labial movement of the lower incisors had been carried out.

The APo line is also used as a guide to facial aesthetics and the latitude allowed for the lower incisor position either side of the line exists for the purpose of permitting the orthodontist to promote the best for the patient's profile, whilst not exceeding the bounds of reason in the matter of post-treatment natural tooth stability.

The NB Line

Some orthodontists prefer to judge the antero-posterior position of the lower incisors before, after and during treatment, and the matter of facial profile, by reference to the NB line rather than APo. This line joins point B and the Nasion and can be used for assessment of labial or lingual movements of the lower incisors in the same manner as the APo line.

As with reference to the APo line, the aim should be, in the majority of individuals, to maintain the original relationship antero-posteriorly of the lower incisor crowns to the NB line in the treated result and not claim unrestricted latitude for labial movement, either by tilting or bodily transference.

When lower incisors are depressed by a plain round archwire and no lower torque auxiliary is used to maintain the long axis angle, the apices will move lingually until they reach the lingual cortical plate. As the apices recede, point B may follow. For this reason the NB line may impose even tighter restriction upon the operator than does the APo line, when the above rule is applied.

Lingual apical or crown movement of the lower incisors seems to be of little consequence to the ultimate stability of the treated condition. It is labial crown movement that should be avoided. Long axis control and root torque to the lower incisors is used to enhance the anchorage value of those teeth and to prevent stultification of their depression through conflict between their apices and the lingual cortical plate, which can occur when free tilt is permitted.

The use of the angle made between the lower incisors and the NB plane as a means of judging a position of stability does not take into account the employment or otherwise of root torque, nor does it give an accurate picture of their true antero-posterior location.

When determining the original position of a lower labial segment relative to the APo or NB lines, reference is usually made to the most labially placed incisor. Should the lower incisors be so imbricated that gross displacement of one has occurred, it would be advisable to base the final positioning of the lower labial segment as a whole, to the lingual, or nearer to the mean, than the displaced tooth.

The Angle SNI

Whereas changes in the position of the lower anteriors in relation to the APo or NB lines are expressed in plus or minus so many millimeters, SNI gives an angular rather than linear means of assessment.

The centre of Sella (S), the Nasion (N) and the incisal edge (I) of the upper or lower incisors, the points forming the angle SNI, are all landmarks which, by cephalometric standards, can be found with assurance, giving little latitude for variable interpretation even by different assessors.

The relative stability of the 'skeletal pattern', as demonstrated by the consistency of angular measurements between one cephalometric plane and another, during the growth of the individual, is well recognized. Volumetric changes occur, producing an increase in the linear dimensions, whilst the general facial morphology remains comparatively unaltered.

The angle SNI has been tested in respect of forty-five growing children through a study of serial lateral radiographs taken annually between the ages of 4 and 12 years. None of the children concerned had received, or was receiving, orthodontic treatment during the period of the study.

It was found that, once the incisors had fully erupted, the angle SNI (upper or lower) showed as little change during growth as any other skeletal angle. Only in four cases did the angle show a gradual change of any significance, but even these needed four years before the alterations became so great they would have upset the reliability of treatment assessment. In other words the angle SNI would provide an accurate means of assessment over an active treatment period of 18 months to 2 years.

A change in the angle SNI of 1° represents a movement of the incisal edge of $1 \cdot 4$ mm in the average 14-year-old patient.

The calculated changes in the upper and lower incisor positions, when using SNI, can be checked back to the original radiograph; for example, if the incisors are now in an edge-to-edge relationship and the changes in the angles SNI indicate a 1 mm retraction of the lower incisors and a 7 mm retraction of the uppers during the preceeding treatment, the original overjet should be found to be 6 mm when measured directly on the original radiograph.

In spite of the apparent accuracy of interpretation provided through the angle SNI, it is advisable in any cephalometric analysis never to trust any one system based on one set of reference points. Cephalometrics, like statistics, offers the opportunity for practitioners to delude first themselves and then others by the ease with which figures can be produced, intentionally or otherwise, which appear to support any contention they may wish to argue. It is therefore recommended that assessment of the lower incisor antero-posterior position is carried out by the use of angle SNI and supported by reference to the APo or NB lines. Each should be found to supply the same answer within a small margin of error.

Tooth Movement Assessment

In order that the measurement of SNI angle reaches its optimum accuracy and/or if further

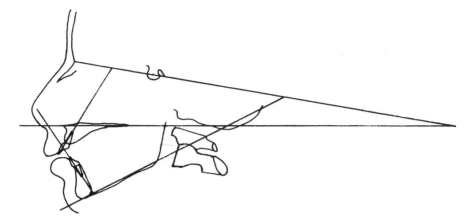

Fig. 6.2. Geometric complex formed by reference lines which can be used for monitoring movement of teeth.

information is sought, for example about the precise amount of incisor apical or crown movement achieved during treatment, additional lines must be drawn onto the lateral skull tracing.

Three horizontal planes, commonly used for reference, recommend themselves both on grounds of convenience and by reason of the comparative accuracy with which they can be plotted on the majority of radiographs: these are SN, the maxillary or palatal and the mandibular planes, or lines.

In addition, lines are drawn connecting the incisal edge and apex of both upper and lower central incisors, thus portraying their long axes. The long axes lines are projected to intersect with two of the horizontal planes which are themselves projected to intersect with each other.

Because the horizontal reference lines may be at times near parallel, it is not always possible to have them intersect within the confines of a tracing sheet of reasonable proportions. When the long axis lines for the incisors are taken in conjunction with the horizontal reference lines, a number of geometrical conformations are produced (*Fig.* 6.2), consisting of straight line intersections, triangles and quadrilateral figures. The angular values, or equalities, of these figures and conformations are matters of simple geometric fact. The angular values, in geometrical terms for the whole of the tracing, should be checked, including, by calculation, angles that would form off the tracing paper. This applies particularly to serial studies over a treatment period where tooth movement is the object of assessment.

In the study of a series of radiographs to determine the extent of tooth movement less error seems to result if the angular figures obtained are geometrically coordinated on the assumption that there is no change in the skeletal pattern. Obviously this applies only to short term studies of tooth movement, not to other forms of study wherein growth changes are, in one form or another, the centre of interest.

Real changes in the angular relationship of the reference planes one to another do take place in some individuals during the growth period, but such changes will be small during any reasonable period of active orthodontic treatment. Faithful attempts to trace what is believed to be there on the radiograph, in respect of the plotting of reference planes, should logically result in the inclusion of genuine growth changes, but this apparent reality can become so inextricably entangled with the falsehoods of inadvertant tracing error, or even be entirely due to it, that tooth movement assessment can in turn become falsified.

Geometric coordination and the use of the above system does not eliminate the possibility of tracing error, but does ensure that the results of the analysis of tooth movement are at least possible, and more accurate than if the method were not used.

It may help to clarify the whole of the above concept if a practical example is given. Tooth movements are not infrequently shown by reference to the maxillary and mandibular planes only. Using this method to analyze cases treated by the Begg technique the long axis changes of the upper and lower incisors can be demonstrated and, in quite a large number of instances, it can also be shown that the angle between the planes of reference has gradually increased over the treatment period, i.e. the maxillary–mandibular plane angle might be found to be 28° at the start of active treatment, 30° by the conclusion of Stage 2 and 31° by the end of Stage 3. The conclusion is drawn that the mandibular plane has been altered by the elevation of the lower molars through the action of the vertical component of force of inter-maxillary Class II elastics. This conclusion is believed because it is logical and therefore in line with what one would wish to believe.

The process of wishful thinking can become disturbed if, in the same case, the line depicting the mandibular plane is projected not only to intersect with the maxillary plane but also with SN. It could well be found that the SN–mandibular plane angle has remained the same throughout the treatment period. This is by no means an unusual finding. The conclusion must be that either the change in the mandibular plane has been compensated for by change at the cranial base, or that the maxillary plane has changed. Closer inspection may reveal that the anterior and posterior reference points, to which the maxillary plane is drawn, have diverged vertically from one another, aided by palatal curvature, so as to produce the alteration in the angle of intersection with the mandibular plane. The orthodontist becomes aware, in this way, of an alternative explanation for the change in the maxillary–mandibular plane angle as a result of the use of dual reference and eventually equally aware that both the frequency and the degree of mandibular plane alteration as a result of Class II elastics is almost certainly less than some may think.

It is not intended to dispute that alteration of the mandibular plane often takes place, but that when it does the change will register against both maxillary and SN planes. Still less is it intended to dispute that mandibular molars are never elevated as a response to Class II traction. On the contrary, reference to the occlusal plane will nearly always show that the mandibular first molars have been elevated and the incisors depressed, resulting in a forward cant of the occlusal plane, but that the movements, including compensatory intrusion of the first upper molar, can occur within alveolar bone and do not necessarily affect the relationship of the basal structures, or alter inter-maxillary height.

The forward cant of the occlusal plane is, at first sight, an undesirable side effect of the employment of the Begg technique. The amount by which the occlusal plane changes during treatment is variable, and dependent upon a large number of factors, including the degree and duration of force application through the Class II elastics and how much of this force has been deployed in the vertical dimension. Orthodontists who employ higher forces are those likely to produce a greater change to the occlusal plane.

When assessing change to the occlusal plane by serial radiographs, much depends on how the plane is represented. If the plane is drawn to the level of the occlusal surfaces of bicuspids and molars, less change will be shown than when the tips of the incisors or cuspids are used for the anterior reference point. Reference to the lower incisor edges would add the intrusion of these teeth to any change in the buccal areas.

Changes to the occlusal plane, as measured by the buccal teeth, are in the region of 1° to 5° and take place during Stages 1 and 2. Some reversion usually takes place during Stage 3 and is completed after appliances have been removed.

The effect of Class II mechanics on the occlusal plane would seem to be transitory and in no way detrimental to the long term success of treatment. It might be added that causing excessive forward cant of the occlusal plane by the use of heavy forces does not necessarily assist successful overbite reduction. Elevation of the lower molar will soon be accommodated by compensatory intrusion of the uppers through occlusal forces.

The Pattern of Tooth Movement, Typical of the Treatment of Class II Division 1 Occlusions, as shown in Serial Lateral Radiographs

In so far as it is possible to depict the tooth movements, occurring during the course of treatment using the Begg technique, through one typical example, *Fig. 6.3* is intended for this purpose. A second similar case, analyzed in *Fig. 6.4*, was also treated by extraction of four first bicuspids, followed by the mechanical Stages 1, 2 and 3, through the standard application of the Begg technique, sometimes called the 'pure' Begg technique. This implies the use of the Begg appliance in conjunction with Class II inter-maxillary elastics as described in the earlier sections of this text and does not include the

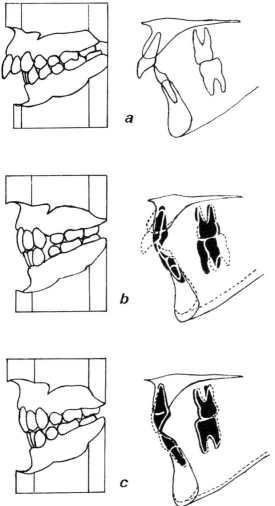

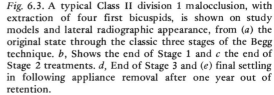

Fig. 6.3. A typical Class II division 1 malocclusion, with extraction of four first bicuspids, is shown on study models and lateral radiographic appearance, from (*a*) the original state through the classic three stages of the Begg technique. *b*, Shows the end of Stage 1 and *c* the end of Stage 2 treatments. *d*, End of Stage 3 and (*e*) final settling in following appliance removal after one year out of retention.

use of extra-oral forces or root torque to lower incisors.

In addition to the classic three stages of active treatment, the illustrations show the important settling in of the occlusion following the removal of the appliance. The word important has been used because the settling in phase is a notable feature of the use of the Begg appliance and arises out of the fact that final tooth placement is not quite so precise as in the use of edgewise. The 'socketing in' of the buccal cusps and the re-establishment of the anterior overbite need not be brought about mechanically but may be left to natural tendencies. An upper removable retainer is used in order to restrain any tendency for relapse of the corrected overjet, whilst the natural vertical adjustments take place, which involves also the restoration of the occlusal plane.

It is mildly amusing to reflect how pleased orthodontists seem to be when an occlusion settles in a manner which accords with their highest hopes and yet, some at least, do not always fully realize that the natural factors that have been at work to give them so much pleasure are the same as those which, on other occasions, have provided them with their greatest nightmare—relapse. Relapse is an unfavourable settling in, settling in is a favourable form of relapse. Which of the two events occurs depends on numerous factors not the least of which is the correct positioning of the treated occlusion within the facial framework.

The molar and incisor movements shown in the lateral skull tracings should not be difficult to interpret, when taken with the explanations offered elsewhere in this text.

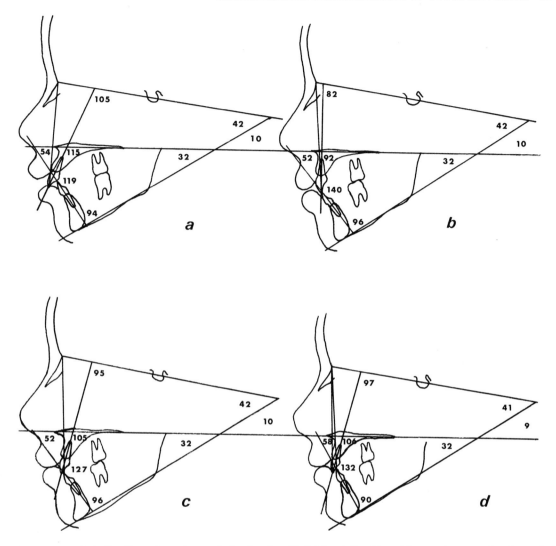

Fig. 6.4. Lateral skull radiograph tracing analysis of a Class II division 1 first bicuspid extraction case, showing typical angular changes as they pertain to the three stages of treatment by the Begg technique. *a*, Original malocclusion: SNIU 82°, SNIL 78°. *b*, End of Stage 2: SNIU 76°, SNIL 76°. *c*, End of Stage 3: SNIU 77°, SNIL 77°. Reference to the angle SNIL, or APo line, indicated that the crowns of the lower central incisors had not been moved labially during Stages 1 and 2. The long axis increase to the mandibular plane, was due to the lower incisor apices being driven to the lingual by the archwire depression force. *d*, Two years out of retention: SNIU 78°, SNIL 77°. After appliance removal the apices reestablish in their former positions as the overbite readjusts. The 1° difference between the SN line and the mandibular plane is the result of a change in the relative angle of SN compared to previous tracings. The change can be real or otherwise, but would be ignored when assessing tooth movement. On the assumption of no change, the upper central incisor long axis becomes 96° not 97°.

Much of the success or otherwise of achieving full overjet reduction and a Class I relationship of the buccal teeth, without spacing in the upper lateral incisor or cuspid region, depends upon the relative success of overbite reduction. This important task is therefore to be the subject of the next chapters and gives the opportunity of discussing certain refinements to the standard Begg mechanics.

The foregoing system of cephalometric analysis is by no means the only one, nor is it complete to serve all purposes for which such systems could be used. Many methods have been devised to assess tooth movement, facial aesthetics, or to promote the needs of research. Downes, Broadbent, Steiner, Ricketts, Tweed, Bjork and Holdaway are amongst the many who have developed cephalometric study for varying purposes.

Attempts to express ideal occlusion or facial harmony in terms of standard statistics, derived from such studies, have perhaps been helpful to students in forming their own ideals. On the whole, however, it is not possible to determine reliably ideal occlusion and still less personal beauty in statistical terms. The statistics have their origin in subjective opinion, a fact which can easily be demonstrated by analyzing the same treatment result by two differing systems. It could well be found that the result harmonizes perfectly with one set of recommended figures, but is somewhat at variance with the other.

In the absence of a really accurate means of individual assessment, before or after treatment, the treatment target tends to be the arbitrary one of producing a Class I relationship; yet everyone recognizes that achieving that objective can sometimes be unwise, sometimes unstable, and sometimes impossible.

Chapter 7

The problem of increased overbite: the prognosis for correction

It is important to the standard of the outcome of treatment that deep overbite, where this is a feature of the occlusion, is eliminated. If this cannot be accomplished for whatever reason, and a proportion of the original overbite persists, full retraction of the upper incisors becomes impossible because of the obstruction offered by the lowers. This in turn means that, where the cheek teeth have been brought to a Class I relationship, space must exist either mesial or distal to the upper cuspids. If this unwanted and possibly unsightly spacing is to be closed, it can only be done by mesial movement of the cheek teeth of the upper arch into a Class II relationship with the lowers, because the desirable alternative of upper incisor retraction is prevented. The continued presence of deep overbite also means that the adjustment of the upper incisor roots by palatal root torque, cannot be carried out without the incisal tips moving labially.

The elimination of deep overbite, where this exists, is therefore the keystone to obtaining the best occlusal relationship. Unless the edge-to-edge, or near edge-to-edge, incisor relationship can be brought about through treatment, the result, from a perfectionist's point of view, must be impaired.

Clinicians would probably agree that successful overbite reduction to the above degree, does not provide great difficulty in the majority of instances, but there does seem to be a minority of cases which do not respond adequately to any of the well tried and usually successful mechanical measures available.

General Observations on Deep Overbite and Prognosis for Correction

Before describing the mechanics for obtaining the optimum in overbite reduction, some general observations follow which aim to illustrate the extent of the overbite problem and the structural variations which collectively supply the cause. In this way the reasons why some cases respond to treatment better than others may become more apparent.

One possible introductory approach to the study of deep overbite and its underlying causes can be through examination of a type of occlusion which provides the orthodontist with no overbite problem, namely cases of Class I incisor relationship. For the purpose of the study the lateral skull radiographs of sixty Class I occlusions in 14-year-old patients were used to provide tracings onto which a series of straight lines were drawn which formed intersections at thirty carefully selected points on the facial skeleton, inclusive of the alveolar processes and teeth. The distances between the points and the angles formed between the lines were recorded, giving seventy dimensions from each tracing.

From the bank of information so collected, it was possible to reconstruct geometrically, with considerable accuracy, the average facial pattern for any sub-group selected from the main sample.

A detailed description of the method would be lengthy and, if given at this point, would deflect from the subject of overbite. Suffice it to say that there are several advantages in such a system. First, through the law of averages, deceptive idiosyncrasies in the facial form of individuals are eliminated and only the strong trends within the group preserved. Secondly, human variations, when studied independently, are often small and when analyzed statistically show little significance from one group to another. The product of small variation, however, can be cumulative and collectively create effects, such as increased overbite, which may well be significant by any standard. The geometric system is capable of supplying readily understandable graphical

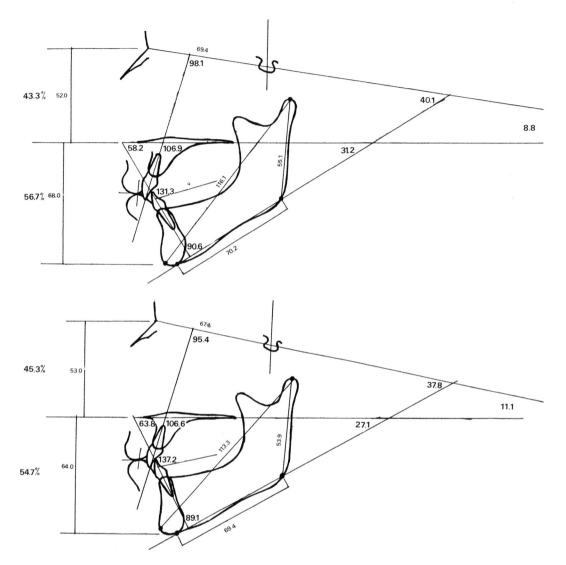

Fig. 7.1 and 7.2. The facial form, reconstructed from average dimensions, derived from lateral skull radiographs, of 30 males (top) and 30 females whose incisor relationship was Class 1. (In all diagrams in this chapter the large numbers are angles, in degrees, the smaller ones measurements, in mm.) All patients were 14 years of age ±9 months at the time of recording. At this age there is minimal difference between the sexes in respect of facial development. [Male: SNA 79·2°; SNB 76·5° (difference 2·7°); total facial height 120 mm; SNIU 81·6°; SNIL 79·6°; average length upper central incisor 26·4 mm; av. length lower central incisor 24·4 mm. Female equiv. data: 78·5°; 76·5° (2°); 117 mm; 80·6°; 78·9°; 24 mm; 22·6 mm.]

information which would be more tedious to render, or comprehend by arithmetic or algebraic means.

Figure 7.1 and 7.2 show the results of reconstruction from averages of the Class sample, when divided equally according to sex (30 males, 30 females). From the full sample of sixty cases, two sub-groups were selected; one containing the

ten cases having the greatest lower facial height (*Fig.* 7.3) and the converse, the ten having the least lower facial height (*Fig.* 7.4). Measurement of facial height was by perpendicular from the maxillary plane to the lower border of the mandibular symphysis. From the superimposition of the average facial forms of the two sub-groups, the influence of mandibular morphology and the

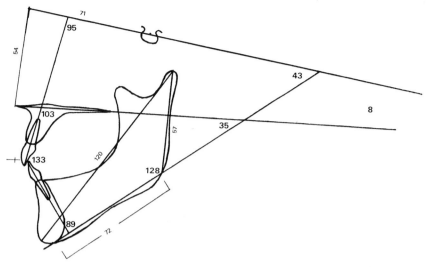

Fig. 7.3. The facial form, constructed from the average dimensions of the 10 cases selected from the main sample of 60 Class I occlusions, as having the greatest lower anterior facial height. [SNA 77°; SNB 75°; lower facial height 73 mm; posterior inter-maxillary height 35 mm; overbite 2·4 mm.]

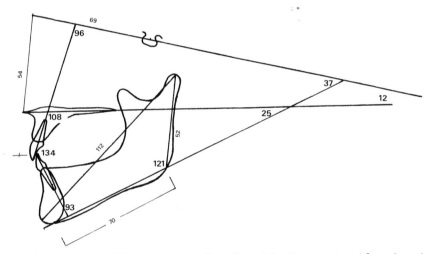

Fig. 7.4. The facial form, constructed from the average dimensions of the 10 cases selected from the main sample of 60 Class I occlusions, as having the least lower anterior facial height. [SNA 78°; SNB 75°; lower facial height 61 mm; posterior inter-maxillary height 28 mm; overbite 4·3 mm.]

relative cant of the maxillary plane on the size of inter-maxillary space, both anteriorly and posteriorly, can be seen (*Fig.* 7.5). The original lateral radiographs were all taken with the teeth in occlusion and not with the mandible in the resulting position, but it has been assumed that the true inter-maxillary space would, in the majority of cases, be closely related to that shown with the teeth in occlusion. It can be seen that, even in groups of Class I occlusion, there might be

considerable difference in the amount of inter-maxillary space which the alveolar processes are called upon to cross.

Current theory is that the inter-maxillary space will continue to be crossed by the alveolar processes and contained teeth, up to the limits of their growth potential, or until obstructed in one of the following ways:

(1) By contact with the teeth of the opposing arch;

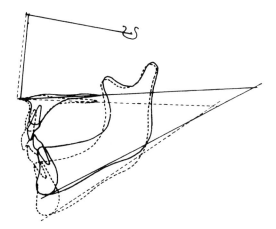

Fig. 7.5. The high lower anterior facial height group (Fig. 7.3) superimposed on the small lower anterior height group (Fig. 7.4) at Sella and on the SN line.

   (2) By contact with the gingival or palatal soft tissues of the opposing arch;

   (3) By contact with the lip of the opposite arch;

   (4) By the intrusion of the thumb or digit;

   (5) By intrusion of the tongue during swallowing and speech; and

   (6) By the presence of a dental appliance.

Where occlusal contact is made between the teeth of opposing arches, prevention of further vertical development is active rather than passive, through the action of the masticatory muscles, which preserve in this way an inter-occlusal clearance between the teeth when the muscles are at rest.

The posterior teeth offer a relatively flat platform against which the forces of occlusion can operate; the incisors, on the other hand, are so shaped and related that they rarely meet edge-to-edge, but by-pass each other by variable amounts, at times failing to contact at all. Consequently, the limiting of incisor overbite through mutual contact will vary in accordance with anatomical form, antero–posterior relationship and the inter-incisal angle.

The presence of a well-formed cingulum on the palatal surface of the upper incisor provides at least a partial platform which can effectively restrain the continued eruption of a lower incisor and is more significant in this respect than the inter-incisal angle, in either the treated or untreated condition. The ideal inter-incisal angle is usually regarded as being in the region of 135°, but

examination of the Class I sample, either individually or in groups, shows that the degree of overbite present is not critically related to the inter-incisal angle.

It is true that acute inter-incisal angles, on average, are associated with the smaller, and the more obtuse with the greater, anterior overbites and that there exists a strong statistical correlation between the two. It would be wrong to deduce, because of these facts, that the one is necessarily the cause of the other. On the contrary, both could be effects produced alike by other soft and hard tissue variations within the facial skeleton which collectively supply the real causes of each.

In continuance of the quest for the real causes of deep overbite, and reverting once again to the Class I sample, there were two cases amongst the ten with the highest lower facial height which had minimal overbites, one of zero overbite and the other showing an anterior open bite of 3 mm. The facial and dental dimensions of these two cases were amalgamated to form Fig. 7.6 and Fig. 7.8 when superimposed at Sella and on the SN line with the high Class I facial group (Fig. 7.3). It can be seen that the group of two cases have an even greater average height to the lower face than the group of ten. The presence of an anterior open bite in persons possessing exceptional inter-maxillary height anteriorly could be due to the distance the dento-alveolar structures have to cross in excess of their potential to vertical development. Such cases of open bite are different to the more usual examples which owe their existence to, for example, the intrusion of thumb or digit. The latter, once the causative habit is broken, readily respond to treatment or resolve themselves unaided. This is not necessarily the case when the open bites are associated with very high lower facial heights. If sprung archwires or vertical elastics, or both, are applied to these cases, results may be disappointing. After minimal initial success, continued application of forces produces mobility of the anterior teeth and perhaps accompanying tenderness. On reduction of the force values, some of the small original improvement is lost, and reversion to the former force values produces the same effects as before. Eventually the project may have to be abandoned. When appliances are removed, the incisors dart back into their sockets. This clinical experience tends to substantiate the theory that the potential to further vertical development of the dento-alveolar

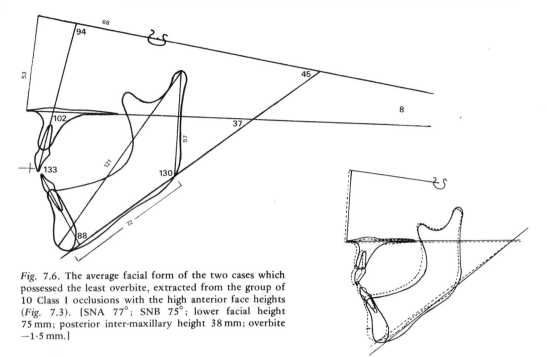

Fig. 7.6. The average facial form of the two cases which possessed the least overbite, extracted from the group of 10 Class I occlusions with the high anterior face heights (*Fig.* 7.3). [SNA 77°; SNB 75°; lower facial height 75 mm; posterior inter-maxillary height 38 mm; overbite —1·5 mm.]

Fig. 7.8. Superimposition at Sella and on the SN line, of the minimal overbite Class I cases (*Fig.* 7.6) upon the average product of the high facial height Class I sample (broken line).

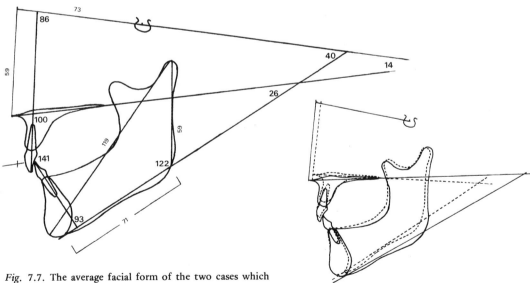

Fig. 7.7. The average facial form of the two cases which possessed the greatest overbites, extracted from the group of 10 Class I occlusions with the heigh anterior face heights (*Fig.* 7.3). [SNA 78°; SNB 74°; lower facial height 68 mm; posterior inter-maxillary height 31 mm; overbite 5·5 mm.]

Fig. 7.9. Superimposition at Sella and on the SN line, of the Class I cases with the largest overbites (*Fig.* 7.7) upon the product of the high facial height Class I sample (broken line).

structures has indeed been exhausted and that the continued use of mechanical forces, far from stimulating further development would, if taken to extremes, result in tooth extraction.

It would seem reasonable to presume that there is a limit to the size of the alveolar structures and that the size, as well as potential, would vary with the individual.

The clinical experience mentioned above which may accompany the use of elevating forces on the anterior teeth will be referred to again when discussing similar force applications to the posterior teeth.

In direct contrast to the two cases of reduced overbite subtracted from the high lower face group of Class I sample discussed above, the two cases having the greatest overbites from the same high facial group were examined. The result of reconstruction from averages of these two cases is shown in *Fig.* 7.7. The two occlusions had been categorized as Class I because clinical appreciation, by itself, gave sufficient grounds for considering any other classification. A glance at the diagram, however, reveals how closely the average of these two individuals approaches the characteristics of occlusions which could almost be classified as Class II division 2. The mild skeletal II jaw relationship is already there and the upper incisors have, on eruption, dropped lingually into contact with the lowers, thereby becoming rather vertically placed; but not crowded, nor sufficiently retroclined, for the clinician to revise his classification. He would unhesitatingly have done so had the lower incisors been placed a few millimeters further to the lingual, which would have allowed some or all the uppers to be guided by the lower lip into a position of more marked retroclination. All that is needed here, for one classification to slide into the other, is 3–4 mm less to the antero–posterior length of the body of the mandible. Alternatively the same situation could be produced if the lower incisors had been held back in a more vertical position by a differing morphology and action of the lower lip, or the gonial angle had been lower, which on average tends to have a similar effect. So long as the upper incisors do not buttress one another through mutual overlap, they will drop back to contact the lowers (*see Fig.* 11.11). The more the latter are to the lingual the greater the opportunity for the uppers to become retroclined to an increasingly marked degree and, incidentally, the higher the inter-incisal angle must become.

It is interesting to ponder upon how little need be the differences in hard or soft tissue morphologies for occlusions to develop which, because of the very existence of the Angle classification, orthodontists are inclined in a reflex way to believe are light years away from each other, but which in reality may be very closely related.

In the Class II division 2 occlusions, variations within the facial form are such that the upper and lower incisors, on eruption, come close to missing one another, or may actually do so. This situation can be produced by many permutations of skeletal, soft tissue and tooth position variations, but, no matter how produced, leaves the incisors free to erupt towards their maximum heights before meeting with obstruction, giving rise to the probability of deep overbite.

Many Class II division 2 and division 1 cases are found to have lower anterior facial heights which are below the average for the same dimension in Class I. One would deduce from this, on the dangerous assumption that vertical alveolar growth potentials are the same in all individuals, that the reduced inter-maxillary space could easily be crossed, with enough reserve potential to continue to do so, as the space becomes increased through growth of the mandible. The deep overbite would therefore persist and show no natural reduction as the patient grew.

In order to demonstrate the circumstances of deep incisor overbite pertaining to Class II division 2, a sample of thirty patients having this form of occlusion have been analyzed in a similar manner to that applied to the sample of Class I occlusion above.

The ten cases having the greatest lower anterior facial height were subtracted from the main sample and their remaining facial characteristics reconstructed from averages, resulting in the form shown in *Fig.* 7.10. The contrasting ten cases, selected from the main sample, which possessed the lowest facial heights are shown in *Fig.* 7.11. When this last diagram is superimposed on the Class I group (10 cases) which had the high lower face, it can be seen by how much small variations in mandibular morphology have allied themselves to reduce the inter-maxillary space both anteriorly and posteriorly (*Fig.* 7.13). *Figure* 7.12 shows the superposition of the group of *Fig.* 7.11 on that of *Fig.* 7.10.

All groups so far depicted can be regarded as within the range of normal variation and will

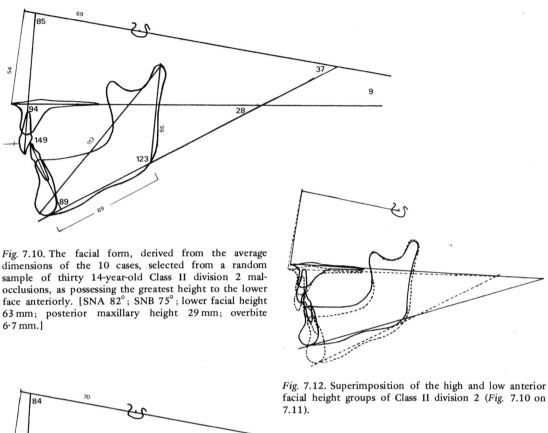

Fig. 7.10. The facial form, derived from the average dimensions of the 10 cases, selected from a random sample of thirty 14-year-old Class II division 2 malocclusions, as possessing the greatest height to the lower face anteriorly. [SNA 82°; SNB 75°; lower facial height 63 mm; posterior maxillary height 29 mm; overbite 6·7 mm.]

Fig. 7.12. Superimposition of the high and low anterior facial height groups of Class II division 2 (*Fig.* 7.10 on 7.11).

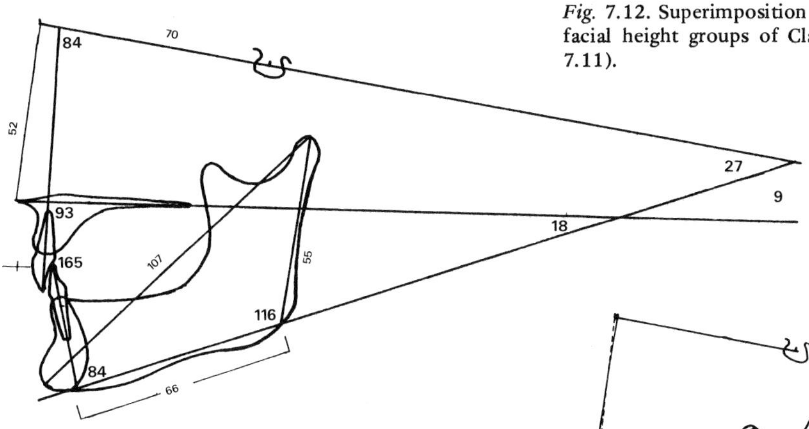

Fig. 7.11. The average facial form of the 10 cases from the Class II division 2 sample with the least height to the lower face anteriorly. [SNA 82°; SNB 77°; lower facial height 54 mm; posterior inter-maxillary height 27 mm; overbite 8·5 mm.]

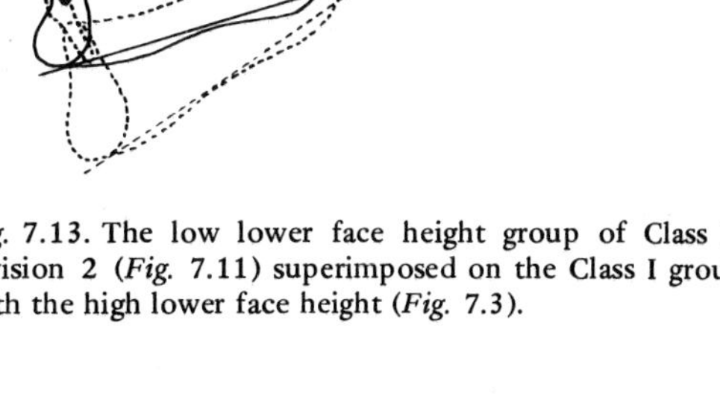

Fig. 7.13. The low lower face height group of Class II division 2 (*Fig.* 7.11) superimposed on the Class I group with the high lower face height (*Fig.* 7.3).

respond to measures of overbite correction, although some amongst the low anterior facial height group of Class II division 2 might respond with difficulty.

Before embarking on a description of extremes in overbite situations wherein mechanical reduction problems are not merely probabilities, but near certainties, it is necessary to draw upon clinical experience of mechanical measures used for overbite reduction in general terms, so that these may be used to augment final conclusions.

General Observations on the Mechanical Control of Incisor Overbite

There are many mechanisms, such as the functional appliances, which aim as part of their effect to control overbite, but, from the point of view of building up a rational explanation for the existence of deep overbite and in attempting to give logical reasons as to why some provide the orthodontist with more difficulty than others, it is necessary to consider only two basic types of mechanical control.

Types of Mechanical Control

Broadly there are two mechanical approaches to the reduction of deep incisor overbite, one passive and the other active. They are:

(1) The anterior bite platform or bite plate; and

(2) The active archwire, often augmented by inter-maxillary elastics or headgear.

The Bite Platform

There is an unusual measure of agreement between researchers as to the manner by which a bite plate brings about a reduction in incisor overbite. The plate has a twofold action:

(i) The presence of the bite platform, against which the lower incisors impinge, arrests the further vertical development of the lower anterior dento-alveolar structure, which would otherwise continue to take place so long as the potential to do so remained. The lower incisor teeth are not, however, measurably intruded by the biting forces. Without intrusion, vertical growth increase alone would only account for, on average, a millimetre or two a year in overbite reduction, through

general growth of the mandible. In fact, bite opening of this proportion is attained, in the majority of cases, in a matter of a few weeks, so long as the appliance is worn with reasonable consistency. The reason for this rapidity of response, therefore, must lie mostly in the second action of a bite plate.

(ii) When the bite plate is being worn, the posterior teeth cannot occlude and are thus relieved of the forces of occlusion. The posterior dento-alveolar processes, under these circumstances, will immediately develop vertically so long as the potential is there, which is usually the case. The effect of this on the anterior overbite is, in all but a small minority of cases, almost immediately apparent and will soon permit adjustments to be made to the inter-incisor relationship in the opposite plane.

The posterior increase in height of the dento-alveolar processes which is encouraged by the bite plate will not, however, become permanently stable until general growth in the vertical dimension has become sufficient to accommodate the increase. If, before this general vertical growth has taken place, the bite plate is removed, the forces of occlusion very quickly re-establish the former occlusal heights of the teeth. Relapse of this kind is experienced when a patient who has been making good progress towards overbite reduction decides not to wear the appliance because, perhaps, of illness. In a week or so all the previous progress is lost. The ease with which progress can thus be lost is a disadvantage arising with the use of a removable bite plate as against fixed appliances.

Most orthodontists will also have come across cases which did not respond to the wearing of a bite platform. Little improvement in the incisor overbite can be detected in these instances, even after months of appliance wearing which is accompanied by irrefutable evidence of the highest standards of patient cooperation. It is not expected that actual incisor depression will be found in conjunction with the wearing of a bite plate, because the patient will, through sensory feedback, discover the precise height and location of the platform during the first twenty four hours of wear. Henceforward, he will avoid biting heavily against the plate in sensible self-defence. What is surprising in these cases is that the usual and expected vertical growth of the posterior segments does not take place. Before attempting to put forward a possible answer to the question of why this is so, further useful evidence can be obtained from clinical experience of fixed appliances.

The Fixed Appliance

Active archwires are capable, unlike the passive bite plate, of causing actual intrusion of either the upper or lower anterior teeth. The amount of intrusion is, however, decidedly limited. As incisors are depressed they become progressively resistant to the forces upon them for that purpose. It could well be that maximum intrusion in either arch does not exceed 4 mm, and might often be less. Once this maximum incisor intrusion is reached, continued overbite reduction, if needed, must be through elevating forces supplied by the appliance to the posterior teeth, assisted by general vertical development of the lower face. The latter factor is both unpredictable and variable and can make possible highly spectacular and unexpectedly good results in some cases, whilst failing to do so in others. In the case of the standard, or pure, use of the Begg appliance, the forces to depress upper and lower incisors are supplied through the anchor bends; but when Class II inter-maxillary elastics are being worn, the intrusive effect of the main archwire on the upper incisors is limited by the vertical component of the elastic force. Posteriorly, the same component of elastic force may cause the extrusion of the lower anchor molars. This elevation of the lower molars will in time be accommodated, either through general vertical growth of the mandible, or by compensatory intrusion of the upper molars through the occlusal forces, or both. At times the extrusion of lower molars can run ahead of the ability of the upper molars to accommodate by intrusion. The result will be a temporary increase in the angle between the mandibular plane and the SN line. This change may not fully resolve until the appliances have been removed.

The comparatively simple mechanics of the pure Begg technique are adequate to handle the majority of overbite problems which are within the range of reasonable variation, but there remain those which are outside that range.

The limited effect of the pure Begg technique on the intrusion of upper incisors, was mentioned previously. In the more difficult overbite situations it may be desirable to modify the technique so that the upper incisors as well as the lowers are intruded to the absolute maximum during an additional treatment stage, and methods have been devised for so doing. The question arises as to whether, if these techniques were applied correctly and to the full, would it mean that the desirable edge-to-edge incisor relationship would be achieved in all cases: the answer is, unfortunately, a firm no.

Cases where Response is Inadequate

It is now necessary to try to explain the nature of the cases that do not respond adequately and to suggest the reasons why.

Every orthodontist will have noticed, clinically, that resistance of the incisor teeth to intrusive forces appears to build up more rapidly when they are housed within an alveolar process which is notably below average height, than when within a bony process of more usual proportions. Alveolar processes of reduced height are found, not surprisingly, in patients whose lower anterior facial height is also reduced by the average standards. A low anterior height to the lower face is a frequent variation, often, but by no means always, to be found in association with Class II division 1 and division 2 occlusions. This feature is frequently, but again not always, allied to a low gonial angle or square mandible, which can be associated with any occlusal pattern, but which is particularly prevalent in Class II division 2.

Another occasional but salutory clinical experience which can attend overbite reduction in Class II occlusions, particularly division 2, is not only to meet with difficulty in obtaining incisor intrusion but also to find, in the same case, that molars do not respond to elevating forces. In the case of the Begg appliance, the inter-maxillary elastics should, with their vertical force component, cause elevation of the lower anchor molars; but in these particular individuals there is little or no such reaction.

Faced with a persistent overbite and an apparent inability to depress the lower anterior teeth or to elevate the posteriors mechanically, it is probable that the orthodontist, in desperation, will slump into a very understandable human reaction; namely, to combat threatened failure by increasing the applied forces. The result is not success, but the creation of mobility of the lower molar teeth, and probably the lower incisors as well.

The similarity between these events in the lower molar region, of mobility without elevation, and those, described earlier, which attended attempts to close anterior open bite in Class I cases with exceptional anterior height to the lower part of the face, is inescapable. It is easier, however, to persuade acceptance of the theory of exhausted alveolar growth potential in cases which can be seen and measured as having a lower face height and dento-alveolar heights of exceptionally large dimensions, than to gain credence for the same hypothesis in cases where the same dimensions are plainly well below the average.

Before proceeding to collect further evidence which might clarify the matter, it should be said that the type of case now under review, whose overbite problems are more than difficult to eradicate, are the same ones that fail in this respect to react to the bite platform, or indeed any other form of appliance.

Looking back at the ten cases with the reduced lower anterior facial heights and Class II division 2 occlusions, the two patients who possessed the greatest overbites were extracted, in order that their collective facial pattern could be examined. The product of the average dimensions of these two individuals is shown in *Fig.* 7.15. *Figure* 7.16 shows the facial form of these individuals when superimposed on the diagram showing the average of the two Class I cases with anterior open bite (*Fig.* 7.6). This gives a good impression of the range of vertical variation of the face and, although the outcome of treatment of the two Class II division 2 occlusions is not known, it also gives an indication of the type of case which might give rise to failure of overbite reduction.

It is not just the amount of the overbite present by which relative difficulty should be judged. Growth amounts and direction are vital in determining the success or otherwise of the applied mechanics, but neither can as yet be predicted with any guaranteed accuracy and a seemingly difficult treatment prospect can, in the event, prove easier than expected. An orthodontist should not despair when confronted by these cases, but should heed the warning.

Patients having the facial form and occlusion of the type shown in *Figs.* 7.14 and 7.15 often have another characteristic, not shown by the diagrams; namely, an unusually large freeway space, or inter-occlusal clearance, when the masticatory muscles are at rest. When the teeth are in occlusion, comparison with cases of normal occlusion shows, on average, an element of overclosure with the mandible rotated forward at the condyle.

Both features could be explained by the belief that the forces of occlusion are greater in these particular individuals than in others, resulting in a depression of the cheek teeth, which brings about both the large inter-occlusal space in the rest position and the overclosure when the teeth are occluded.

If the occlusal levels of the teeth are established through the occlusal forces alone, the question recurs as to why the consistent wearing of a bite plate, giving relief from those occlusal forces, fails to promote adequate response in certain individuals (*see* p. 66). Why is it that, in the same cases, active elevating forces to the posterior teeth fail to promote vertical development of the alveolar processes and are liable instead to produce looseness of the teeth?

It is difficult to avoid the conclusion that natural vertical growth does not take place; nor can artificial forces stimulate the event, because the required growth potential is simply not there. Acceptance of such an answer means accepting also that there must exist a considerable range of variation in alveolar size, and that this is, largely, genetically predetermined for each individual.

If the dento-alveolar heights in the mandibular arch were to be so predetermined, the differing levels and curvatures of the occlusal planes formed in different individuals would be explained. Once the level of the mandibular teeth is set, the upper alveolar process and contained teeth would grow to meet the lower, so long as there existed the potential to do so. Any failure of such a capacity would mean that the mandible would need to be overclosed in order to obtain occlusal contact.

It does seem to be the case that the contribution made by the upper alveolar process to the crossing of the inter-maxillary space is greater in some individuals than others, and this is most noticeable anteriorly. It may even be that the greater upper anterior alveolar heights, when associated with a lip morphology which fails to provide adequate camouflage, contribute to that unfortunate feature picturesquely called the 'gummy smile'.

Occlusal forces probably do little more than prevent unwanted vertical growth of the alveolar processes. That such forces can depress teeth whose occlusal levels have been artificially raised

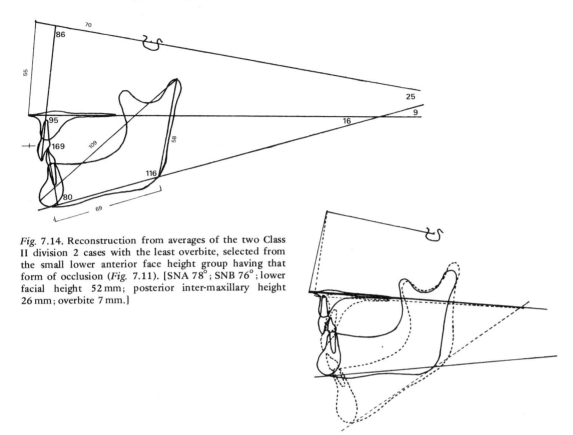

Fig. 7.14. Reconstruction from averages of the two Class II division 2 cases with the least overbite, selected from the small lower anterior face height group having that form of occlusion (*Fig.* 7.11). [SNA 78°; SNB 76°; lower facial height 52 mm; posterior inter-maxillary height 26 mm; overbite 7 mm.]

Fig. 7.16. The two greatest overbite cases from within the low face height group of Class II division 2 (*Fig.* 7.15) superimposed on the average of the two minimal overbite cases of Class I (*Fig.* 7.6).

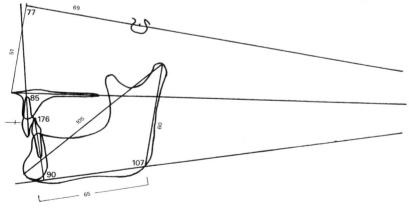

Fig. 7.15. The two cases with the greatest overbite, selected from the low lower anterior face height group of Class II division 2. The angles off to the right are: SN–maxillary plane 8°; SN–mandibulary plane 17°: min–max. 9°. [SNA 82°; SNB 76°; lower facial height 50 mm; posterior inter-maxillary height 24 mm; overbite 11 mm.]

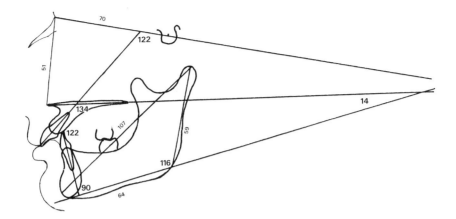

Fig. 7.17. Individual patient with a Class II division 1 malocclusion, having a similar facial form to that shown for division 2 in *Fig.* 7.15. The angles off to the right are SN–maxillary plane 12°, and SN–mandibular plane 26°. [SNA 77°; SNB 77°; lower facial height 54 mm; posterior inter-maxillary height 28 mm; overbite 10 mm.]

by, for example, the fitting of overlays, is beyond question; but does not necessarily mean that this ability is used in normal developmental circumstances.

Whatever may be the truth of these arguments, it would appear probable that, where a measure of failure to reduce overbite occurs, it is due to an inadequacy of growth rather than to the orthodontist or his appliances.

Not only must growth quantities be adequate, but also growth directions. The Class II division 2 facial pattern shown in *Fig.* 7.15 can be compared to an individual example of Class II division 1 (*Fig.* 7.17) and the similarities in general facial morphology noted. It would not be surprising to find that these patients all showed mandibular growth of the closing rotation pattern, whereby posterior inter-maxillary space increased disproportionately to the anterior. This is the reverse of what the orthodontist would like if incisor overbites are to be eliminated.

It can be seen from the diagrams and descriptions that the occlusions which threaten difficulty in overbite reduction are often associated with a low gonial angle, amongst other features. It should perhaps be said that a low gonial angle is one of the commonest ways by which anterior facial heights can become limited, so contributing the possibility of severe overbite. Its mere presence, however, is no guarantee of that possibility, nor is the square mandibular angle the only variation which can produce a low anterior facial height.

Some Class II division 1 occlusions achieve the same low anterior face height by possessing a mandible of well below average size in all dimensions, but with an average gonial angle. These cases too can be overbite reduction problems, because intrusion of the upper and lower incisors even to the maximum possible extent, may still be inadequate where overbites are severely increased. Growth alone can solve the problem.

Where mechanical measures and accompanying growth fail to eliminate an overbite, there is nevertheless always some improvement. Upon the degree of that improvement will depend the standard of the compromise treatment result.

The Influence of the Soft Tissues

Finally, to complete the incisor overbite picture, examples should be given of the influence of the soft tissues in either permitting or limiting this feature. These effects are best seen in Class II division 1 occlusions and are not usually associated with any mechanical difficulty.

Using a sample of twenty Class II division 1 cases, and applying the same mode of group analysis used for Class I and Class II divison 2, five cases within the main sample showing incomplete overbite were withdrawn, and their average dimensions used to construct *Fig.* 7.19. For comparison, five cases having complete incisor overbites were withdrawn from the same sample and their averages treated in the same manner,

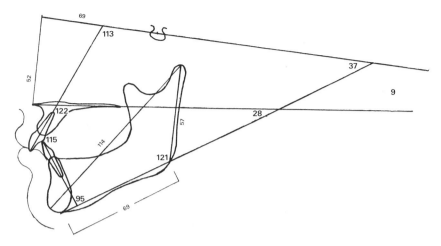

Fig. 7.18. Reconstruction from the average dimensions of 5 cases of Class II division 1 malocclusion, having complete anterior overbite. Selection was from a random sample of 20 Class II division 1 14-year-old patients. [SNA 81°; SNB 79°; lower facial height 61 mm; posterior inter-maxillary height 28 mm; overbite 6·8 mm.]

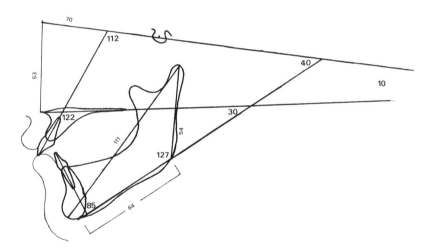

Fig. 7.19. Reconstruction from average dimensions of 5 cases of Class II division 1 malocclusion, having incomplete overbite, taken from the same sample as used in *Fig.* 7.18. [SNA 78°; SNB 74°; lower facial height 61 mm; posterior inter-maxillary height 27 mm; overbite 1 mm.]

resulting in *Fig.* 7.18. The lip morphologies associated with these cases have been drawn in to show the limiting effect the lower lip might have on the full eruption of the upper incisors.

Both groups have an identical anterior facial height, but, in the case of the incomplete overbite group, there is less tissue to the upper lip, contributing to lip incompetence. In these cases the patient swallows by using the tongue above the tips of the lower incisors and against the lower lip, in order to provide an anterior oral seal.

By so doing the space between the upper and lower anteriors is perpetuated and a decrease in overbite maintained. It would seem probable that it is the existence of a space between upper and lower incisors which triggers the swallowing behaviour, rather than the latter forcing the tooth positions. The complete overbite cases whose average is shown in *Fig.* 7.18 have a lower anterior dento-alveolar height exactly equal to the Class I average, when measured from the lowest point on the mandibular symphysis to the lip of the lower central incisor. The incomplete cases (*Fig.* 7.19) show a measurement for this structure which is 2 mm below the Class I average. Both measurements are compatible with the form and dimensions of the mandibles concerned and the summit position of the red margin of the lower lip. The latter feature being invariably closely coordinated with lower dento-alveolar height.

Conclusion

In so many of the foregoing thoughts and arguments the orthodontist faces the old question of which came first, the chicken or the egg—or in some instances, eggs. It would be a pleasure to have the answers scientifically proved beyond doubt. Many of the facts are available; but the difficulty lies more in their interpretation than with the facts themselves.

Chapter 8

The problem of increased overbite: the mechanics for correction

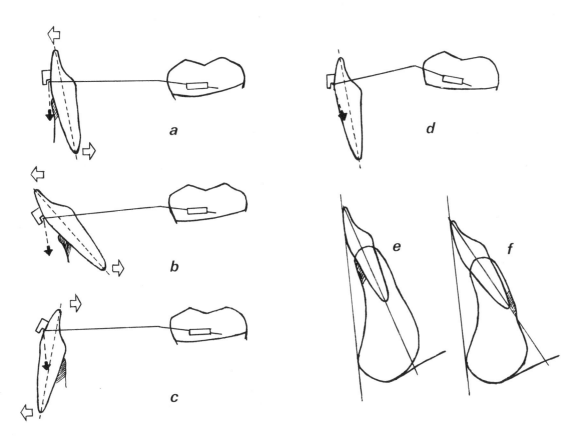

Fig. 8.1. The direction of the intrusive force from a main lower archwire relative to the long axes of the lower incisors.

a, The usual situation wherein the force, not quite in line with the long axes, promotes a labial crown movement which is resisted by the labial cortical plate of the investing bone. The result is lingual movement of the root ends until slowed by contact with the lingual plate.

b, The reaction shown in *a* will be more positive when the lower incisors are markedly labially inclined initially and the supporting bone section wide.

c, The initially upright or lingually inclined lower incisors. In this instance the intrusive force promotes further lingual tilt and, through the support of the lingual cortical plate, labial root movement.

d, Vertical and horizontal relationships between the anterior and posterior teeth and appliance attachments can alter during Stage 1, so that the reaction shown in *a* can become changed to that shown in *c*. This, allied to the effect of toe-in bends as they work their way through the distal of the molar tubes, together with minor local factors, can cause actual retraction of the lower anteriors during Stage 1.

e and *f*, The areas of resistance of labial crown movement and lingual root movement to the tilting response of lower incisors to an archwire intrusive force.

In the use of the standard, or pure Begg technique, increased anterior overbites are reduced by the combined mechanical effects of the anchor bends and the vertical component of force of the inter-maxillary elastics. The incorporation of anchor bends causes the upper and lower archwires to lie well into the mucco–buccal fold anteriorly, so that once pinned into the bracket slots of the incisors, intrusive forces are created.

The inter-maxillary elastics, through their vertical component of force, produce not only elevation of the lower molars posteriorly, but also have a similar effect on the anterior of the upper archwire. The latter fact is not conducive to upper incisor intrusion, in that it cancels, or partially cancels, the intrusive force of the archwire in that region. It follows therefore, that if upper incisor intrusion is to be sought at a level of maximum possibility, the standard technique for the use of the Begg appliance, must in some way be modified.

It will also be recalled, from the descriptions in previous chapters, that the intrusive force of the lower archwire, when applied to lower incisors which are usually labially inclined before treatment, causes an accompanying increase in the long axis angle of these teeth relative to the mandibular plane. The angular increase is almost wholly attributable to the lingual movement of the root apices of the lower incisors, with little associated labial movement of the incisal edges. The pivotal point for this movement is near the necks of the incisors, a fulcrum being provided by the presence of the labial cortical plate (*Fig.* 8.1).

The resistance of the labial plate means that the tips of the lower incisors should seldom be found labial to their original relationship to the APo line, at the conclusion of Stage 1.

During the closure of any residual extraction space, carried out in Stage 2, the lower incisor crowns will be retracted away from the inner aspect of the lower lip, although the long axis increase produced during the previous stage may not become fully corrected.

The amount of the increase in the long axes of the lower incisors to be anticipated during overbite reduction, is dependant to an extent upon the cross-sectional shape and size of the alveolar process in which the teeth are contained. The limiting effect of the lingual and labial cortical plates means that less labial tilt can be expected for lower incisors contained within a narrow

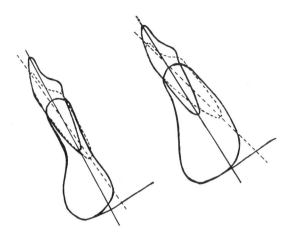

Fig. 8.2. Intrusion of lower incisors. Force delivered by a plain round archwire to incisors, already labially inclined, will cause lingual displacement of the apices which will be greater for those individuals with a wide alveolar process opposite point B than for those with a narrow. Mechanical control may be needed to prevent excessive tilt and keep the depression force more in line with the long axes of the teeth.

isthmus of bone than for those in a wider one (*Fig.* 8.2).

In the case of a narrow cross-section of bone, labial tilt may be controlled, but the mechanics of the appliance will nevertheless still be promoting that movement, resulting in continuous pressure between the roots and the cortical plates. This is a situation productive of bone and root resorption, which feature has indeed been demonstrated in this particular area and circumstance (*Figs.* 8.3 and 8.4).

The wider the alveolar process in the region of the lower incisor apices, the better the prospect of rapidly promoting an excessive amount of long axis change, so that the lower incisors become markedly angled across the process early in the overbite reduction procedure and before the desired edge-to-edge situation has been reached. Indeed, it is often the case that, where the bony process is wide, the lower incisors have a marked labial inclination at the outset; and, if there is scope for their apices to move further to the lingual, the application of the appliance will soon have this effect, so that the direction of the intrusive force becomes progressively further from the long axes of the teeth and the teeth themselves become so angled that they become wedged between the cortical plates, rather than being driven down the centre of the bone. This situation

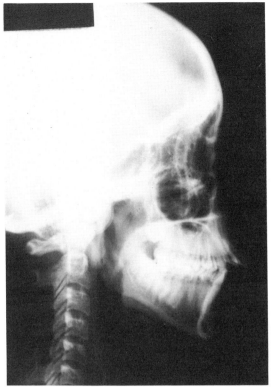

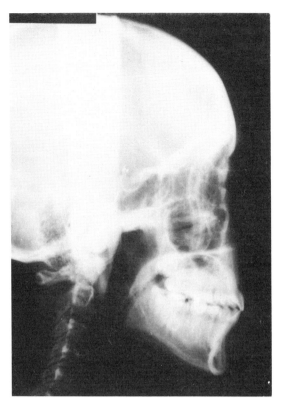

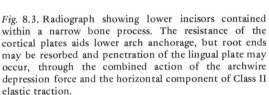

Fig. 8.3. Radiograph showing lower incisors contained within a narrow bone process. The resistance of the cortical plates aids lower arch anchorage, but root ends may be resorbed and penetration of the lingual plate may occur, through the combined action of the archwire depression force and the horizontal component of Class II elastic traction.

Fig. 8.4. Radiograph of the same patient as shown in *Fig.* 8.3 at the conclusion of active treatment, showing lingual displacement of the lower incisor apices. This displacement can be expected to relapse with regeneration of the lost bone.

would logically reduce the success and extent of continued incisor intrusion and a means of prevention must therefore be devised.

Arising out of the foregoing observations, it becomes necessary to describe mechanical measures which are supplementary to the basic and which aim to improve both the control and extent of overbite reduction using the Begg appliance. It should perhaps be said that the measures to be described relate to the more obdurate of overbite problems, or where the disadvantageous factors, outlined above, apply. The reduction of incisor overbite in the more usual circumstances can still be effectively accomplished using the standard Begg technique, and any attendant root resorption should be minimal if force application is kept suitably light.

Long Axis Control of Lower Incisors During Intrusion to Reduce Overbite

In order to minimize root resorption, prevent premature angling of the lower incisors across the alveolar section with attendant threat of penetration of the lingual plate by the root apices, coupled with the possibility of labial movement of the incisal edges, it may be desirable to apply a modest amount of labial root torque during the action of incisor intrusion.

The application of labial root torque will have the effect of uprighting the lower incisors over basal bone, bringing the incisal tips away from the lower lip and their apices away from the lingual plate, at the same time placing the teeth in a more vertical position, which ensures that the direction of the intrusive force is more in line with their long axes. Theoretically, this means greater mechanical efficiency with less damage to the roots and the removal of the possibility of premature stultification of the full intrusive effect. It would also mean that there would be some justification for the use of labial root torque routinely when depressing lower incisors.

From the practical point of view, there is the desirability of keeping to simplicity of method unless, through a more complex means, real rather than theoretical advantage can be gained.

In the case of a narrow alveolar process, the control given by the buccal and lingual cortical plates will be such that the lower incisors cannot tilt more than a minimal amount. If root torque is to be used in this circumstance, it would be less for the purpose of maintaining uprightness and more as a means of avoiding resorption of the roots through pressure between them and the cortical plates. There is no doubt that such resorption can take place, as elsewhere in the mouth when continuous pressure is sustained, keeping root apices in contact with lingual, labial or palatal plates of bone. The heavier the pressure the more likely the loss of tooth tissue and/or penetration of the plate. What, at the present time, is not quite so clear, is whether the application of root torque causes a reduction of apical loss of practical significance as against the use, in the same situation, of the standard Begg technique. More evidence is needed.

If the root penetrates the cortical plate, the apical position can be expected to relapse later, accompanied by regeneration of the bone.

The above observations relating to lower incisors within narrow bony confines would also apply where the bone width is average, although the slight increase in width would permit more labial tilt if labial root torque is not applied. In the average case, adequate bite opening without apical loss can usually be achieved by the standard Begg technique, the lingual displacement of the apices reverting as the proper overbite reestablishes following the removal of the appliances. This is not an argument against the use of root torque, but rather an observation that it might not always be necessary.

Where the lower alveolar process is exceptionally wide and in particular the contained incisors are markedly labially inclined before treatment, the intrusive force from the main archwire will produce the maximum degree of tilt, because of the direction of force relative to the long axes of the teeth and the absence of control from the labial and lingual plates. In addition to displacement of the lower incisor apices lingually, some labial movement of the crowns may be anticipated. The process is liable to be rapid and progressive.

The mechanical effect of a plain archwire is inefficient in such circumstances, being productive of tilt rather than intrusion. The application of some labial root torque provides long axis control, thereby improving effectiveness of intrusion and preventing the crowns of the lower incisors from wandering towards the lower lip.

Two forms of torque auxiliary were illustrated in *Figs.* 5.10 and 5.11, but in the context of Stage 3 of treatment. It remains to comment on their application to Stage 1.

In case of possible confusion, it should perhaps be said at this point that there is a subtle difference between the purpose of labial root torque to lower incisors as used in Stage 1 and that for the same arrangement in Stage 3. The purpose of a root torque auxiliary in Stage 3 is to finalize apical positioning bucco–lingually, where one or more were, or have become, misaligned and at the same time, to increase to total anchorage value of the lower arch. In Stage 1 the purpose is to facilitate proper intrusion and minimize apical loss. This latter purpose should already have been achieved by the commencement of Stage 3.

If the two auxiliaries previously described are now put into a Stage 1 context, the first (*Fig.* 5.10) can be regarded as an efficient but somewhat clumsy arrangement. Oral hygiene is not easily maintained whilst the auxiliary is being worn. The fact that it is ligated into place and that the superior aspects of the multiple loops rest over the tops of the brackets introduce the possibility of occlusal interference from the upper incisors in situations where overbite has not yet been fully reduced.

The design of the second auxiliary is more appropriate to the avoidance of possible occlusal interference and more conducive to the maintenance of proper standards of oral hygiene.

When either auxiliary is used in the context of Stage 1, the wire forming the auxiliary should terminate just posterior to the lower cuspid brackets. There are some who choose to extend the free ends of the auxiliary so as to enter the buccal tubes alongside the main archwire and others who extend to the distal of the second bicuspid brackets. What may be lost by so doing is the efficiency not of the labial root torque, but of intrusion. It is difficult to make two identical archwires and activate them to produce an identical intrusive force. If the attempt is made and the archwires fitted into the buccal tubes side by side, one wire is bound to interfere in some measure with the efficiency of the other. Extending the auxiliary to engage the brackets of the second bicuspids will also limit effectiveness of intrusion of the lower anteriors and is inadvisable for Stage 1 procedures, although it might be added that in Stage 3, after intrusion has been already carried out, extension to the second bicuspids would become appropriate.

It may be necessary, in Stage 1, to carry out preliminary alignment and levelling of the lower incisors before the torquing auxiliary, of whichever pattern, can conveniently be fitted.

In the interests of simplicity and of saving time and chairside effort, it would seem desirable to avoid the use of a supplementary or auxiliary archwire. This implies a need to redesign the main archwire in order to bring about both active depression and labial root torque simultaneously through the same wire. *Figure* 8.5 shows a lower archwire design for the above dual purpose.

The angle of the gate sections to the plane of the archwire will be dependent upon the initial long axis angle of the lower incisors. The more proclined these teeth, the greater will be the angle between the gates and the plane of the archwire. The torque force should be felt as the fitting sections of the wire are brought into the bracket slots, but should be only just positive enough to be detected, with no great amount of effort needed to insert the archwire into the slots of the brackets. An advantage of the use of the 0·018 in wire rather than 0·016 in is to minimize the risk of introducing slight rotations to the lower incisors, but this is probably more of a theoretical than a practical consideration. With suitable adjustment, force application should not vary whichever gauge is employed.

The arguments against this form of torquing arch can be expected to arise from adverse experiences gained from the use of similar methods in the upper arch in the days when spurs were bent into the main archwire rather than an auxiliary.

When vertical spurs were bent into the main archwire for the purpose of palatal root torque to upper incisors, it was found that, as the spurs were

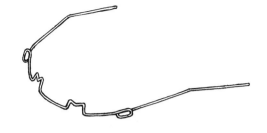

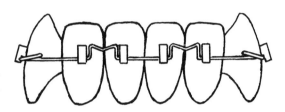

Fig. 8.5. Lower archwire for labial root torque. Barely perceptible torque of only a few degrees is sufficient to supply long axis control against labial tilt of lower incisors during active intrusion. The spurs are M-shaped to facilitate adjustment to fill the inter-bracket span and assist avoidance of occlusal interference.

placed in position and the archwire fitted into the bracket slots, the torque was transmitted to the horizontal sections of the archwire, causing any incorporated bends or loops to rotate and the posterior of the archwire to expand across the molar region. Anchor bends and traction loops no longer remained properly orientated and, during treatment, the inter-molar width was increased.

Before discarding the lower archwire pattern on the grounds that it would have the same disadvantages, certain essential differences should be pointed out.

In the days when palatal root torquing spurs were bent into the main upper archwire, it was advocated that the spurs should be set to form an angle of 25° between themselves and the plane of the archwire. The torque force resulting would be potent, particularly in cases of marked upper incisor retroclination. The greater the amount of torque applied to the incisors, the greater the amount of rotation in the buccal aspects of the wire when fitted and the greater the amount of posterior expansion which can be anticipated.

In the lower arch, the amount of torque required to maintain the roots of the lower incisors away from the lingual plate is small. Consequently, the amount of archwire rotation in the buccal regions when pinned into the incisors is also small and does not affect the orientation of the anchor bends or traction loops to a degree having practical significance. Expansion created across the molar region is likewise slight and, in any case, would merely augment a posterior expansion normally built into a lower Stage 1 archwire. This pattern of archwire can be of particular value in the treatment of some bimaxillary protrusions (*see* chapter 14).

Supplementing Vertical Anchorage to Assist Incisor Intrusion

The vertical anchorage available from the first permanent molar teeth is adequate for successful incisor overbite reduction in the majority of cases. There remain the minority which possess overbites of exceptional depth, the most obdurate being often associated with adverse skeletal form and patterns of mandibular growth.

In such cases resistance to intrusion of the incisors can build up quickly against the force supplied through the anchor bends. It follows that if the anchor bends remain active, but meet resistance from the anterior teeth, their continued activity can still produce movement elsewhere, namely in the molar region. The anchor molars will begin to tilt distally with a rise of the mesial marginal ridge and a commensurate depression of the posterior. The lower anchor bends will gradually become closer to the buccal cusps of the upper teeth and will be more exposed to subsequent damage from occlusal forces. In short a situation will develop which is highly undesirable, both to the security of the appliance and its effectiveness.

It becomes desirable to increase the resistance of the first molars against distal tilt if further intrusion of the anterior teeth is to continue. Many appliance techniques achieve this effect by banding the second permanent molars and extending the main archwire to attachments on these teeth. The inclusion of the second permanent molars gives support against possible tilt of the first (*Fig.* 8.6*c* and *d*).

As mentioned in chapter 4, the use of the second molars is not easily accomplished with the Begg appliance, without upsetting the concepts of the conventional mechanics of that apparatus.

As a substitute, or alternative, to the banding of the second molars, the Begg appliance can be used with posterior vertical elastics. In order to support

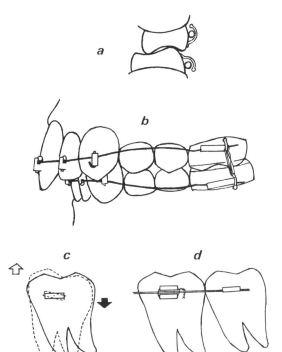

Fig. 8.6. *a* and *b*, The use of posterior vertical elastics to hooks on the disto–buccal aspects of the upper and lower first molars as a means of offsetting the tendency of these teeth to tilt distally under the influence of the anchor bends. The system shown can be augmented by inclining the buccal tubes slightly towards the gingival and keeping the anchor bends near the anterior of the tubes.

c, The molar tilt tendency in reaction to the anchor bends which increases in proportion to the resistance of the anterior teeth to intrusion.

d, The use of the second molar to assist vertical anchorage by aiding resistance to first molar tilt.

the distal of the first molars against depression, vertical elastics can be applied to the distal of the upper and lower archwires as they emerge from the buccal tubes (*Fig.* 8.7). The wires must be turned so as to form a suitable hook, or the elastic may be shed. Direct application of the elastics to the archwires interferes to an extent with the archwire function and free sliding capacity. As an alternative, it has been suggested that the elastics should be applied to vertical hooks, curved around the buccal tubes and fitted towards the distal of the first molar bands (*see Fig.* 8.7*a* and *b*).

If the desired intention is to attempt continuation of lower incisor intrusion only, Class II inter-maxillary elastics can be continued in conjunction with the posterior vertical elastics, but if

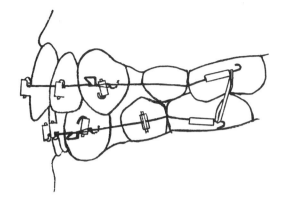

Fig. 8.7. The application of vertical posterior elastics to the ends of the main archwires. The effect is to supplement the depressive force on the incisors, whilst decreasing the leverage from the anchor bends on the molars, by relieving archwire contact at the distal of the buccal tubes.

reinforcement of the posterior anchorage is to assist upper incisor intrusion as well as lower, the Class II mechanics must be suspended until the overbite becomes sufficiently reduced. This amounts to a separate Stage 1 bite opening phase, which, once accomplished, is followed by the conventional Stage 1 procedure.

Severe overbite problems, such as might demand the additional mechanics outlined above, are most commonly found in Class II occlusions, particularly division 2. The latter form of occlusion tends to have a reduced height to the lower third of the face and alveolar processes which are also reduced in height vertically when compared to the Class I average. In addition, some or all the upper incisor teeth are retroclined. In severe cases of this type of occlusion, it has been suggested that the separate bite opening phase be combined with upper palatal root torque. An upper anterior root torque auxiliary is fitted to take the apices of the upper incisors palatally and away from the floor of the nose into an area where further intrusion can be contemplated. In this way the occlusion is early transformed into Class II division 1 with reduced overbite. Once this stage has been achieved, the Stage 1 mechanics proper are started. The same introductory mechanics also overcome another problem of some Class II division 2 occlusions, namely a shearing or scissor incisor relationship which would threaten to strip off any brackets placed on the lower incisors. Once the upper palatal torque arch is fitted, the upper incisor

crowns will respond by moving labially so clearing the labial surface of the lowers for the placement of brackets.

Perhaps the greatest difficulty inherent in the use of any of the foregoing supplementary mechanics is in knowing which cases need such measures and at what point in treatment they should be applied. This is due to a further difficulty which underlines so many other issues; the uncertainty of growth prediction. The orthodontist is aware of severe incisor overbites, associated with what appears to be a mandible of unfavourable morphology from the point of view of the probable pattern of future growth, which nevertheless responded to treatment through the normal Begg technique unaided by supplementary mechanics. Retrospective assessment invariably reveals that success was due to growth vectors which were wholly favourable, in spite of original appearances.

A separate bite opening stage, consuming time and effort, should not be embarked upon unless it is strictly necessary. Rather than lay down any rule of thumb it is probably preferable to allow orthodontists, knowledgeable of the facts at issue, to act in accordance with the observed response to treatment in each individual case.

The Use of Headgear for the Purpose of Overbite Reduction

At a risk of being accused of unnecessary repetition, it might be again mentioned that the use of Class II mechanics in the Begg technique partially obliterates the effectiveness of the upper anchor bends to intrude the upper incisors. The discontinuation of the inter-maxillary elastics and the fitting of posterior vertical elastics reinforces the anchorage for the depression of both upper and lower incisors, but does interupt, in a sense, the general continuity of treatment progress.

There are circumstances, involving the need to intrude the upper labial segment, where yet another mechanical alternative could at least be considered.

The alternative is the use of extra-oral anchorage by the application of high pull headgear to the anterior of the upper archwire to assist the intrusion of the upper labial segment. The use of headgear is not part of the basic Begg technique but is worthy of consideration in particular individual cases.

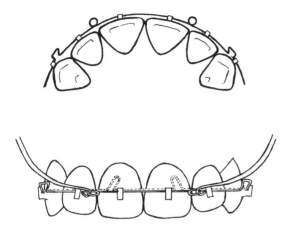

Fig. 8.8. Occlusal and anterior views of main upper archwire with additional rings for the receipt of straight or high pull headgear. The possible simultaneous use of a spurred torque auxiliary for palatal root movement is indicated by the broken line. Some compression of the anterior segment of the main archwire can be anticipated from the headgear force and observation kept for any molar expansion.

The type of case in question will most probably be of the Class II division 2 classification where the standard application of Stage 1 of treatment has induced the maximum depression of lower incisors either attainable or desirable, but left the upper incisors insufficiently intruded from the same points of view.

High pull headgear can be used to finalize upper incisor intrusion, attachment to the anterior section of the archwire being to additional traction rings placed between the upper central and lateral incisors, Fig. 8.8. The archwire should be of either 0·018 in or 0·020 in gauge, in order to provide strength against possible distortion from the headgear forces. The latter should be kept light by the standards of extra oral forces, i.e. approximately 250 g.

Note should be taken, when depressing upper incisors, of the position of the central incisor apices relative to the nasal floor. In cases showing greatly increased incisor overbite, the lower facial height is often below average and the heights of the alveolar processes similarly reduced, leaving little bone above the apices into which to intrude.

In the Class II division 2 occlusions it may be necessary to accompany upper incisor depression and retraction with the use of light palatal root torque from a spurred auxiliary, so that the upper incisors apices can be eventually intruded into an

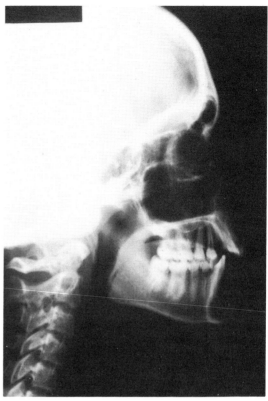

Fig. 8.9. A Class II division 1 malocclusion before treatment. The upper alveolar process is narrow and the position of the palatal wall may severely limit the repositioning of the upper incisor apices, following crown retraction.

area of more copious bone. Again note must be taken initially of the shape and location of the palatal wall, because the existence of this barrier will arrest palatal root movement (Fig. 8.9).

Once upper incisor intrusion has been accomplished, there will be little difficulty in sustaining the situation through the standard Begg mechanics. Class II elastics, worn during the period of the use of high pull headgear, should be kept light around 50 g pressure and worn during day time. The headgear is worn, without the Class II mechanics, for the nocturnal hours.

High pull headgear can also be applied to Class II division 1 cases for the same purpose and in the same manner as above; but it is probable that, due to the upper incisor long axis angle relative to the direction of force application, no palatal root torque will be required.

The use of high pull or, in the face of lost

mandibular anchorage, straight pull headgear, does not invalidate the Begg technique. The mention is made as a reminder of the existence of extra-oral anchorage which could be used in conjunction with the Begg appliance either in an emergency, or to cover the existence of the unusual.

One form of emergency could be the premature expenditure of mandibular anchorage, through mechanical error. Some use of headgear could avert the need to supply anchorage through further extractions.

The unusual will include the cases of severe overbite, discussed above; but these are by no means the only representatives of the unusual. Malocclusions do not always present for treatment as some form of average. Teeth may have already been extracted which one might well, from an orthodontic point of view, wish to have still been present. Teeth may be congenitally absent where one would wish them to be present. Eruption may be delayed of teeth which would otherwise have provided useful anchorage. Occlusions exist wherein it would be undesirable to extract in either the bicuspid or first permanent molar regions but where extractions, if needed, should be of the second permanent molars, both in the interests of the standard of result and the time taken to achieve it.

It is easy to forget the problems set by these anomalies when discussing appliance procedures in general terms. The Begg appliance must be made to supply these mechanical needs by suitable addition or modification to the basic technique so as to cover the unusual, as well as the usual, in the varied demands of tooth movement programmes, if it is to survive into the next generation.

Chapter 9

Factors influencing the choice of units for extraction: the effects of differing extractions on appliance mechanics

So far attention has been focused upon the mechanical elements of the Begg appliance, their composition at each stage of treatment and the technique employed to obtain the desired results. For clarity it has been presupposed that the first bicuspids have been extracted in all instances. It was thought advisable to keep these descriptions free until now, of discussion of diagnostic criteria. As a result, nothing has so far been said of the reasons for extraction, apart from the general justification based on the theory of Stone Age man's attritional dentition. Plainly, even if it is considered that this theory makes the extraction of some teeth obligatory in all instances, it does not automatically imply that the units to be removed must be the first bicuspids. More consideration must therefore be given to the necessity or otherwise of extraction and to descriptions of any alteration to technique, or appliance mechanics, which result from the choice of units for extraction other than first bicuspids.

The Necessity of Extraction

The displacement of individual units from the dental arch, or their rotation, is commonly associated with a lack of space for their accommodation in proper alignment. The situation of general overcrowding can be tackled in one of two ways. Firstly, in cases of minor tooth displacement due to lack of space in the supportive structures, the dental arches can be enlarged through antero–posterior or lateral expansion, or a combination of the two. Alignment of the teeth will be brought about, but there is always a lurking fear that success may not be permanent. Permanency of the treated result will not only depend on the new relationship of teeth and a mutual support given through their points of contact, but also on growth suitably enlarging the area of tooth support so as to provide space to permit stable accommodation of the teeth in their new positions. If growth enlargement is inadequate, some measure of relapse can be expected. Fear of relapse following dental arch expansion in minor tooth discrepancy cases is always countered, in the mind of the orthodontist, by the fear of creating too much space if he should resort to extraction. This latter fear can be shown to be very real, particularly in cases which show subsequent growth enlargement greater than predicted. Faced with this dilemma, many orthodontists have adopted, in the border line case, the safety first tactic of treating initially on non-extraction principles, with a subsequent unretained period to test natural stability. Extraction of selected units will be undertaken for those individuals for whom this test has failed.

For teeth to be moved to new positions and subsequently to remain there without artificial aids demands more than just appliance therapy; there must be an attendant accommodating change in the balance of the natural environment through growth and, in the case of the soft tissues, maturation. Growth alone is seldom sufficient to compensate for any but the milder degrees of overcrowding.

Where overcrowding is more marked, the

second option must be brought into play; namely, extraction for the provision of space. Extraction alters the balance by reducing the size of the dental arches to coordinate with the size of their supporting structures, whereas expansion methods rely on the supporting structures enlarging to accommodate the full dentition.

Choice of Teeth to be Extracted

The teeth commonly preferred for extraction are the first bicuspids, because the choice provides the orthodontist with mechanical advantages which frequently help to minimize overall treatment time by providing an anchorage balance more advantageous than would be the case with alternative choices. Extraction of the first bicuspids divides the dental arches fairly equally, leaving the labial segments intact whilst, at the same time, leaving the most teeth possible in the posterior anchorage. This situation allows immediate use of the extraction space for retraction and/or alignment of the labial segments, and facilitates adjustment of anterior overbite. Extraction further posteriorly in the buccal regions diminishes posterior intra-oral anchorage, whilst increasing demand on that anchorage wherever labial segments need to be retracted. It can be anticipated therefore, that the removal of the second bicuspids will result in the provision of slightly less space for the alignment of the anteriors than would be the case with the loss of the first. The space created for the anteriors will be slightly further reduced if the first permanent molars are preferred for extraction. On the other hand, the removal of the first permanent molars provides more space posteriorly for the eventual accommodation of third molars than the extraction of bicuspids.

The advantage of symmetrical extraction is that subsequent mechanical interaction is the same for both sides of the mouth in all but a few atypical circumstances. This balanced mechanical action reduces risk of actively producing asymmetry or centre line displacements.

Before deciding that the maximum anchorage advantage created by the extraction of the first bicuspids make their removal the choice for all seasons, certain issues should be put forward.

First, the situation of maximum anchorage advantage is not always suitable for cases which can be foreseen as demanding little in respect to posterior anchorage, for example, occlusions

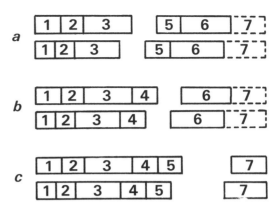

Fig. 9.1. The balance of posterior versus anterior anchorage following the extraction of first bicuspids (a) second bicuspids (b) and first permanent molars (c). It is obvious that the further posteriorly the extractions are performed, the fewer teeth in the posterior anchorage and the more in the anterior, altering the balance of horizontal anchorage; but perhaps less immediately obvious is that the balance in the vertical dimension will also be affected. The units have been diagrammatically expressed by different size rectangles as a reminder of their differing anchorage values; cuspids and molars being the most resistant. Exact quantification is not possible because of innumerable associated variable factors. Relative root area, although involved in the equation, is but loosely related to anchorage response.

devoid of or possessing minimal overjets and/or minor overcrowding of the arches. Extraction of the first bicuspids in such circumstances is liable to bring about a prolonged space closure stage (Stage 2) and induce at the same time, even with the use of the facility of reversal of anchorage, the possibility that the dental area of the patient's profile will become unduly flattened to the detriment of general facial appearance. It would be more appropriate, and less time consuming in the circumstances, to leave more teeth anteriorly and fewer in the posterior region so that the balance of anchorage favours closure of space more from the posterior of the arches than the anterior. In other words extraction, if needed at all, should be in the second bicuspid or even first permanent molar region for these individuals. The exact prediction of the effects of differing anchorage balances created by differing extractions upon the mechanical outcome is an important piece of knowledge which must come to each orthodontist largely through his or her personal experience. Books or journals can be expected to give little more than guidance in principle (Fig. 9.1).

Two different orthodontists, treating near identical occlusions and utilizing the same appliance technique, can nevertheless expend differing amounts of intra-oral anchorage. When this fact is more specifically related to employment of the Begg technique it can be said that some of the more experienced and competent operators find that the anchorage economy inherent in the standard use of the appliance is so great, in their hands, that they come to prefer extraction of second bicuspids, rather than first, in a higher percentage of cases than many of their colleagues. It would be good advice, however, to those beginning with the Begg appliance, not to assume mastery until they can prove it and to create space by extraction which will not make subsequent anchorage control critical.

It must also be realized that one cannot always have a completely free hand in the choice of extraction. For example:

1. There may be teeth congenitally absent, or space may exist as a result of previous extraction carried out for reasons other than orthodontic;
2. Teeth, other than those of primary choice for extraction, may be carious beyond recall, or have been so extensively restored that doubt is raised as to their long term future;
3. Teeth may be so misplaced and/or buried, that there is no practical prospect of repositioning them by orthodontic means and/or in a reasonable period of time; or
4. Individual units can be malformed, or be incompletely calcified, or exhibit internal resorbtion.

When one or more of the above items are exhibited within a case for orthodontic treatment, space may already exist, or have to be created, in locations which may, or may not, be appropriate to the anchorage balance of the required tooth movements. It will be up to the orthodontist to judge whether or not, in the enforced circumstances, he will be able to reach a conclusion which will satisfy his own conscience and be acceptable to the patient without indulging in any further extractions, or without extending the overall treatment period beyond the tolerance of the patient's goodwill. The situations created by missing teeth or enforced extraction can be, plainly, many and varied and therefore virtually impossible to cover by detailed example and instruction. The orthodontist must draw on his experience and knowledge of basic principles to think through the treatment programme, together with any variations which may be needed to the conventional mechanical approach.

The ability to come to the correct conclusions in these awkward and atypical situations, is as important as the mastery of appliance techniques. There is usually a way out of difficulties created by missing units, even though the space given is not exactly where one would wish it to be, but innevitably there will be situations where the location and/or amount of space, is so unfavourable to the subsequent handling of intra-oral anchorage, that further extraction may become the basis for the only hope of ultimate success. This is one of the ways by which a 'multiple extraction' situation can be produced.

Some Implications of the Extraction of Second Bicuspids to the Appliance Mechanics

If second bicuspids are preferred to the first for extraction there will be no call for any fundamental change to the application of the standard Begg technique. The main difference will be in the alteration to the balance of anchorage. In Class II cases, the upper first bicuspids will be added to the load of overjet reduction, thereby increasing the demand on lower posterior anchorage, whilst, at the same time, depriving the latter of the support of the lower second bicuspids. In consequence, it can be anticipated that less space will be obtained anteriorly after the demands of anchorage have been met through the extraction of the second bicuspids than through that of the first.

Where second bicuspids have been extracted, the first can be left unbanded initially in most instances, without detriment. The upper first bicuspids can tilt freely whilst, in the lower arch, the intrusive effect of the anchor bends can act directly on the lower labial segment without the resistance of the first bicuspids being added. It might be advisable in this and other equivalent situations where the lower archwire is left unsupported in the buccal regions, to step the archwire gingivally, in order to obviate the possibility of damage to the unsupported spans from the cusps of teeth in the opposing arch during mastication (*see* Chapter 3). The necessary small vertical adjustment bends must be sufficiently posterior to the lower cuspid brackets to permit lower incisor alignment, unless this has already been accomplished. The posterior adjustment bend must not interfere with the anchor bends, nor obstruct the controlled mesial movement of the molars. Following the reduction of overbite and overjet, the first bicuspid bands are added and any residual extraction space closed by the usual Stage 2 methods.

The above approach, however, should not be regarded as an immutable rule. The banding or bracketing of the bicuspids is a matter for judgement in the individual case. There will be occasions when initial displacement or rotation of the bicuspids may interfere with, for example, the freedom of the upper segment, from left 4 to right 4, to be retracted because of cuspal obstruction. Under such and similar circumstances, the bicuspids must be brought under control early and bands and brackets fitted to them. This will ensure their early alignment and vertical height adjustment with the teeth of the labial segments. Once alignment has taken place, the presence of brackets on the upper first bicuspids should not prevent smooth retraction of the whole of the upper labial segment, but the bracketing of the lower first bicuspids may be disadvantageous to continued overbite reduction, should it be needed.

The fact that the lower bicuspid brackets will, at the onset of treatment, usually lie below the level of the incisors or cuspids, mean that the first stage aligning will adjust occlusal levels by intruding the teeth of the lower labial segment whilst elevating the first bicuspids. Thereafter, the anchor bends combined with the relatively low position of the molar tubes will continue, slowly, the arch levelling process and, in the case of average overbites, may establish the desired edge-to-edge incisor relationship.

The inclusion of the first bicuspids by full bracket engagement with the main archwire, however, effectively adds these teeth to the anterior vertical anchorage. This means that, once levelling has taken place, the anchor bend is active on the molar and reciprocally, primarily on the first bicuspid bracket, in the manner of a 'gable roof' bend. The first bicuspids must be intruded along with the labial segment, which will place more strain on the molar anchorage. The anchor molars may, in consequence, begin to show, not only continued elevation, but a distal tipping. In patients where simple arch levelling is insufficient to obtain full overbite reduction, the above situation can arise and may call for the use of posterior vertical elastics as described in Chapter 7.

It may also be of assistance, where bicuspids are fully engaged with the archwire, to decrease the posterior anchor bends, but, at the same time, to incorporate small vertical bends at intervals along the length of the archwire. In practice this amounts, in the lower arch, to supplying a general curvature to the archwire in the opposite direction to the curve of Spee. The same action can be taken in the upper arch, where the curvature will be seen as an exaggerated curve of Spee. The object of incorporating increased or reverse curvatures is to relieve the molars of some of the anchorage load resulting from incisor intrusion by including bicuspids in this responsibility.

The method is employed not only to continue overbite reduction but also to assist keeping the overbite, once reduced, from relapsing as in Stage 3 archwires previously described. Further examples will be given in association with first permanent molar extraction and non-extraction cases, where bicuspids may at times also need to be fully engaged with the main archwires.

The Extraction of First Permanent Molars: Effects on Treatment

In spite of the fact that the first permanent molar is the larger tooth than either of the bicuspids, it is a practical fact that their removal provides less space for the alignment of the anterior teeth than the extraction of four bicuspids. This is due to the anchorage balance set by the nature and extent of the tooth movements which are likely to follow first molar extraction. All teeth, from second bicuspid to second bicuspid, lie anterior to the extraction sites and only the second permanent molars remain to the posterior. The latter thus become the sole suppliers of posterior anchorage on a reciprocal intra-oral basis. If there happens to be much overcrowding and/or need for retraction of the teeth of the anterior segments, available anchorage may be at a premium.

It should be realized that, whatever the theoretical potential may be for the retraction of cuspids and bicuspids into the space created by first molar extraction, the practical distance that can be achieved is limited, not so much from a lack of anchorage, as by the time factor.

Using the Begg appliance, cuspids and bicuspids will be retracted at first by tipping. If these teeth initially appear to be mesially inclined with the root apices well to the distal, the situation is favourable to the greatest amount of retraction of the crowns by tilting, which could mean near a unit of retraction either side by the time the distal inclination of the second bicuspids has reached maximum. Once this maximum has been reached, any further retraction will have to be a bodily one, which will put more stress on time and anchorage. Subsequent correction of the tilting will also have the same effects.

In less favourable cases, where the cuspids and bicuspids are more upright, or actually distally inclined, prior to retraction, the onset of the need for bodily movement will arrive earlier, possibly before a full unit of retraction is reached. Treatment time will be increased in proportion to this bodily movement factor.

For these practical reasons it comes about that the space released through first molar extraction for the anterior teeth is limited but, because some two-thirds of the extraction space will have to be closed by the mesial movement of the second molars, the unerupted third molars will be provided with more space than would have been the case following the choice of bicuspid extraction.

It is seldom that the anchorage balance offered by the extraction of first permanent molars is so suitable for the treatment of any given case that they become the teeth of prime choice for removal. More often, prior neglect has led to premature loss of one or more of these teeth, or they have been subject to extensive restoration, giving rise to reasonable doubt about their long term future. If the restorative work is of good quality, extraction should not be automatic. Clearly there is cause for considering heavily restored teeth as candidates for extraction where such is needed, but in the case of first permanent molars, prior thought must be given to the likely standard of the outcome of treatment and the overall time factor, bearing in mind the observation of some cynics that the removal of first permanent molars, as opposed to other units, halves the standard of treatment result, whilst doubling the time taken to achieve it. This is an exaggeration, but from what has been said earlier, it can be realized that there is an element of truth in it.

The Begg appliance handles the situation following the removal of first permanent molars at least as well as any other current form of fixed appliance and, in the opinion of many, better. The reasons for the comparative success lie in certain inherent qualities of the Begg appliance, namely:

1. The use of lighter forces than those associated with effective application of other appliances, in conjunction with:
2. The facility to reposition the crowns of the teeth early by simple tipping; and
3. The efficiency of the Begg uprighting springs in correcting the roots of the tipped teeth, whilst making comparatively modest demands on anchorage (*Figs.* 9.5, 9.6, and 9.7).

Appliances which employ brackets, with horizontally placed slots, and an archwire to control the long axes of cuspids and bicuspids during retraction, seem to demand more time and anchorage for the treatment of first molar extraction cases than does the Begg appliance.

In order to describe the technique for the use of the Begg appliance in the treatment of first molar extraction cases, it is helpful to divide the treatment prob! s broadly into two categories:

1. Where the individual teeth do not show great displacement or rotation, but where the prime objective of treatment is the reduction of an overjet or bimaxillary protrusion; and
2. Where the incisor teeth are normally related, both in respect to inter-incisal angle and angle to base, but where the buccal teeth are well forward in relation to the incisors with consequent labial prominence of the cuspids.

Obviously these two occlusal formations can be encountered within one individual, for example, where the upper arch conforms to the pattern of the first category and the lower to the second in a Class II division 1 relationship. Although other permutations exist, it is not necessary to mention these in order to demonstrate appliance technique.

Treatment Example *a*

The first hypothetical case chosen to illustrate treatment technique using the Begg appliance after extraction of first permanent molars, is one in which both dental arches conform to the description in category 1 above. The general alignment of the individual teeth is good, with minimal signs of overcrowding, but no spacing is present except in the extraction sites. There exists an increased incisor overbite and an increased overjet, with the cheek teeth in a Class II relationship (*Fig.* 9.2a).

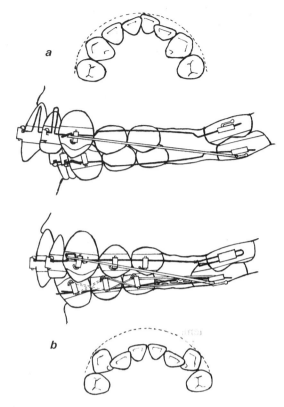

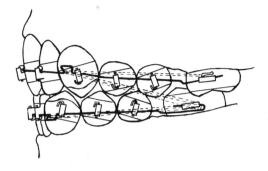

Fig. 9.3. Stage 2 mechanics for final space closure for first molar extraction case.

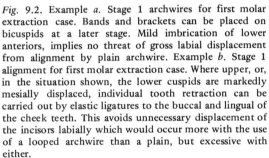

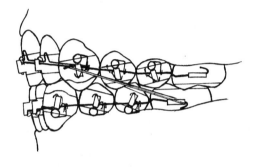

Fig. 9.4. Stage 3 mechanics for the first molar extraction case. In the illustrations covering Stages 1, 2 and 3 of first molar extraction mechanics differing forms of molar control have been shown. They would not, however, necessarily be used in the contexts depicted.

Fig. 9.2. Example *a*. Stage 1 archwires for first molar extraction case. Bands and brackets can be placed on bicuspids at a later stage. Mild imbrication of lower anteriors, implies no threat of gross labial displacement from alignment by plain archwire. Example *b*. Stage 1 alignment for first molar extraction case. Where upper, or, in the situation shown, the lower cuspids are markedly mesially displaced, individual tooth retraction can be carried out by elastic ligatures to the buccal and lingual of the cheek teeth. This avoids unnecessary displacement of the incisors labially which would occur more with the use of a looped archwire than a plain, but excessive with either.

The main treatment objectives will be to reduce overbite and to retract all the upper teeth anterior to the extraction sites into a Class I relationship with the lowers, using Class II inter-maxillary elastics to the lower second molars as anchorage. These latter teeth will be moved forward into the lower extraction spaces, whilst the upper second molars are controlled against mesial drift during the first stage of treatment. These requirements are all directly in line with the tooth movements derived from the application of Stage 1 of the standard Begg technique.

Once the Stage 1 tooth movements have been carried out, some space may still exist in the extraction sites. These can be closed by the conventional Stage 2 methods, which should result in a slight over-retraction of both labial segments in order to compensate for the foreseeable forward shift of the dental arches during Stage 3 root repositioning (*Fig. 9.3*).

It is probable that, in Stage 3, few if any of the teeth anterior to the extraction sites will require mesial apical movement. Cuspids and bicuspids will be distally inclined to variable degrees (*Figs. 9.4, 9.5*). The leverage supplied through the distal movement of these roots (*Figs. 9.6, 9.7*) will cause the dental arches to move labially and this effect will be further enhanced by any palatal root movement of the upper incisors. Only the second molars can counter the general forward arch shift, through the bodily control given to them by the anchor bends. One might expect, with such an

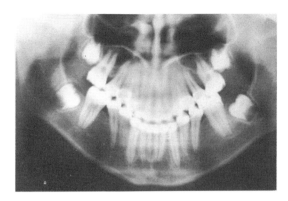

Fig. 9.5. Radiographic appearance at the commencement of Stage 3 of a first molar extraction case, showing the distal inclination of the buccal teeth.

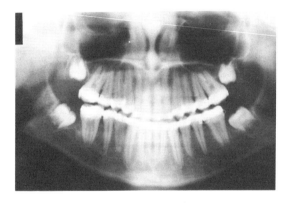

Fig. 9.6. Root movements are relatively slow by any appliance. This is the case shown in Fig. 9.5 after eight months use of root-paralleling springs.

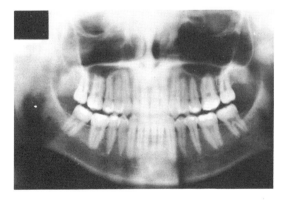

Fig. 9.7. The same case two years after appliance removal. Root movements tend to be more stable than crown repositioning after discontinuation of retention.

unfavourable balance of reciprocal apical anchorage, that the amount of forward shift of the dental arches might be greater than usual in these instances. This does not, however, seem to be the case in practice, where the amount of forward movement is rarely found to exceed the usual 2–3 mm.

Additional anchorage support can be supplied, where needed, to the lower incisors in Stage 3, by the fitting of a labial root torque auxiliary of the type and manner of application described earlier (Fig. 5.11). As always in Stage 3, it is important to ensure that the extraction spaces cannot reopen.

Although it would appear that the straightforward application of the three classic stages of the Begg technique would supply all that is needed for the treatment of the present example, certain additional issues must be raised, since they can cause some modifications to the appliance in first molar extraction cases.

It will be recalled that the extraction of the first molars induces a situation wherein the second permanent molars have to be moved mesially, on average, some two-thirds of the extraction sites, before contact will be gained with the second bicuspids. The second molars, due to their root anatomy and the extent of the surrounding bone buccally and lingually, show a greater tendency to lingual roll when moved along a round archwire by inter- or intra-maxillary elastics, than do first molars. This tendency is all the greater if the second molars are markedly lingually inclined before treatment is begun. The obtaining of the maximum anchorage value and the avoidance of lingual roll, or mesio–lingual rotation, of the second molars is a prime mechanical reoccupation in treatments where the first molars are absent and much of the space remains to be closed.

Various methods have been suggested, or recommended, of improving control of the second permanent molars against lingual roll and rotation:

1. The use of buccal tubes which are oval in cross-section, rather than round;
2. The use of round tubes of conventional size in conjunction with a recurved archwire;

and, from the standard use of the Begg appliance:

3. Expansion of the main archwires across the molar region, particularly the lower; and
4. The application of the inter-maxillary elastics to lingual cleats or hooks on the lower second molars, instead of the more frequently employed hooks on the buccal.

Each of these measures is worthy of a critical appreciation as to their individual merit.

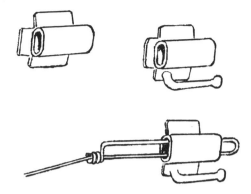

The Oval Tube

The fitting of oval tubes, rather than round, to the second molars enables a measure of increased control to be obtained against lingual rolling by the insertion of a double archwire (*Fig.* 9.8). The archwires are recurved from their distal extremities and brought anteriorly to the position of the anchor bend, at which point the free end is wound round the main archwire. The two wires should lie parallel with each other and the doubled section must slide freely within the oval tube. Due to the long unsupported section of archwire crossing the first molar extraction sites, coupled with the relative instability of the wound-on means of terminating the redoubled section, the anti-roll control given to the molars is not great.

Fig. 9.8. The oval buccal tube and redoubled archwire as a means of stabilizing the molars against lingual rolling.

A combination of posterior arch expansion together with some active lingual root torque, applied through the redoubled section, assists the effectiveness of anti-roll control, but may also introduce frictional resistance within the tube. Watch must consequently be kept on the lower labial segment to see that it does not move labially as the lower molars move forward, arch length having been inadvertantly maintained by frictional binding.

The upper second molars show far less tendency to roll and root torque can be avoided in the upper arch and with it any frictional binding, which would be disadvantageous to incisor retraction.

The general stability of the recurved sections is further improved if the wire gauge used is 0·018 or 0·020 in. The use of larger gauge working archwires, rather than 0·016 in. has other advantages yet to be discussed, in the first molar extraction case.

One problem which can arise from the use of the oval buccal tubes concerns their size compared to that of the standard round tube and the difficulty which can sometimes be experienced in fitting them to the lower second molars. The vertical space on the buccal of the lower second permanent molars, particularly those already lingually inclined, can be so restricted that oval tubes cannot be accommodated without the cusps of the upper second molar impinging upon them. The use of the smaller dimension round tubes becomes virtually enforced. This does not mean, however, that the anti-roll mechanism of a double

archwire cannot be used, but rather that the manner of application must be modified.

The Standard Round Buccal Tube and Recurved Archwire

Where the use of round buccal tubes has been enforced, or is the preferred alternative to oval tubes, archwire control against lingual molar roll can still be imparted through doubling the archwire in the molar region.

The archwire will be doubled back at its distal extremities in the same manner as that used with the oval tubes, but it will not be possible to introduce the double section from the mesial of the tubes. The archwire will have to be inserted from the distal of the buccal tubes, with the main section lying outside and to the gingival (*Fig.* 9.3). The manner of insertion means that the recurved section cannot be wound on to the main archwire, but this makes little if any practical difference to general stability if 0·018 in. wire is used. The mechanical control obtained is essentially the same as provided by the oval assembly, previously described.

The recurved section should not terminate within the tube if friction is to be minimized: enough wire must be left to the mesial of the tubes to allow the molars to be moved mesially a few millimetres and still avoid the free ends of the archwire entering the lumens. On the other hand, if too much free wire is left, insertion of the archwire may become difficult.

As with the double archwire in oval tubes, so with the recurved wire in round tubes: the recurved section should deliver slight lingual root torque to the lower second molars which may give rise to some frictional resistance, as a result of which the lower labial segment should be watched for signs of labial crown shift.

Using the recurved archwire, the effects usually obtained from the anchor bends are supplied by adjustment at the posterior loops. If these loops are opened so as to cause the main archwire and the recurved section to diverge from each other, the main archwire anteriorly will lie in the buccal sulcus when the subsidiary arms are in the buccal tubes. The main archwire, when elevated to the mouths of the anterior brackets, should be found to deliver the same force value as would be desirable from conventional anchor bends. The archwire will lie to the gingival of the buccal teeth which will assist incisor depression and keep the archwire free of opposing cusps. Buccal height adjustment bends are required, if the archwire is to be engaged in the bicuspid brackets.

Toe-in can also be supplied through adjustment of the recurved section of the archwire which enters the buccal tube, by bending the free end slightly in a buccal direction at the posterior loop.

The above double archwire system, like that employing oval tubes, is far more frequently used for the control of lower second molars than uppers. The upper second molars can nearly always be controlled by the conventional anchor bend and toe-in mechanism in conjunction with an 0·018 in. archwire placed in standard round buccal tubes.

It can be added, at this point, that those with some experience of the Begg appliance, find that they can usually control lower second molars by the same conventional means and with the same gauge archwire, resorting to double archwires only occasionally, when necessity demands, rather than as a routine.

An advantage of fitting round tubes rather than oval, in the first instance, is that conventional archwires can be fitted and used throughout treatment or, if somewhere along the line it can be seen that the second molars are beginning to roll lingually, the second type of recurved archwire mechanism described can be fitted without having to change the buccal tubes.

Expansion of the Posterior of the Main Archwire

The practice of maintaining expansion on the posterior of the main archwires across the molar region, as described earlier for the standard Begg technique in association with bicuspid extraction, is also applicable to the first molar extraction case. The expansion helps to counter lingual roll and more will need to be applied to the lower arch than the upper when standard Begg archwires are being used.

The posterior of the recurved, or double, archwires should also be kept expanded, but the amount may need to be reduced if lingual root torque is being applied to the molars. Part of the torque action will be to move the crowns of the second molars to the buccal.

It would almost certainly be unwise to state the specific amounts of either molar root torque or archwire expansion which should be applied, since tooth movement response varies, as does the exact nature of the case under treatment. It would be sounder advice to suggest that these adjustments should err on the conservative side at first and increase gradually thereafter as circumstances dictate. The arch expansion will be reduced as the molars are moved forward, so becoming less in Stage 2 and eliminated in Stage 3.

Application of Inter-maxillary Elastics to Lingual Buttons or Cleats

The transference of the Class II elastics from the lower molar buccal hooks to buttons or cleats on the lingual surfaces changes the direction of the forces to elevate the lingual rather than the buccal and to cause slight expansion rather than contraction across the molar region, whilst continuing to supply the antero–posterior force component. It would therefore seem to be a satisfactory arrangement to counter lingual molar roll.

In the case of the second permanent lower molars, the use of lingual elastics may retard the rate of lingual molar roll but is seldom, if ever, sufficient for correction. The explanation would appear to be that the buccal elevating component of force from the main archwire is greater than that from any reasonable inter-maxillary force from an elastic, so that some molar roll may still take place, even when the inter-maxillary elastics have been transferred to the lingual.

The application of the inter-maxillary elastics to the lingual side of the anchor molars will augment the anti-roll action of the combination of posterior archwire expansion and lingual root torque from a double or recurved archwire and

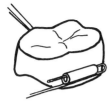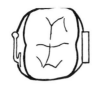

Fig. 9.9. Application of inter-maxillary elastic to lingual hook to assist correction of mesio–lingual rotation, or augment lingual root torque, initiated by suitable adjustment to the redoubled archwire.

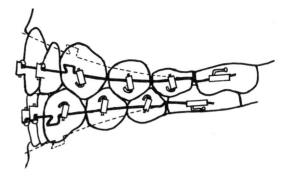

Fig. 9.10. Use of increased curve of Spee in the upper archwire and reverse curvature in the lower to maintain reduction of incisor overbite when bicuspids are fully engaged with the archwire.

will assist their effects to a greater extent than when the inter-maxillary elastics are used with a conventional archwire (*Fig.* 9.9).

The Banding of Bicuspids: The Use of Archwire Curvatures, Corresponding to Increased or Reverse Curves of Spee

In cases where the bicuspids happen to be well aligned, not rotated, nor in need of separate retraction, treatment can be initiated without bands and brackets on these teeth. The depression forces from the anchor bends can then act directly upon the anterior teeth without the intervention of the bicuspids. The omission of bicuspid bands in these particular circumstances is not a rule but an option. If the option is taken, there will be a long span of unsupported archwire between second molar and cuspid which could be liable to damage. It must be seen that there is no threat to the integrity of the lower archwire from the cusps of the opposing teeth. If the threat exists, the archwire must be stepped out of the way of occlusal forces using small vertical bends (*Fig.* 9.2*a*). The bends must be so positioned that incisor alignment is not obstructed and the action of the anchor bends not altered.

The use of 0·018 in. archwires, rather than 0·016 in. aids resistance to potential damage and also affects force application. Because of the probability of considerably increased length of the archwires, in the first molar extraction case, the force for intrusion of the labial segments from a given size of anchor bend in 0·016 in. wire would be lighter than if the same size bend and gauge of wire were used for a shorter archwire applied to the first molars as anchorage. It would be necessary therefore, where second molars are supplying the anchorage, either to increase the size of the anchor

bend in 0·016 in. wire, in order to promote the required force anteriorly, or alternatively to increase the gauge of the archwire. The use of 0·018 in. or 0·020 in. wire, enables the anchor bend to be kept to modest proportions, whilst still supplying, over the increased span, the ideal force for incisor depression.

For those who prefer to band the bicuspids as early in the treatment procedure as possible, or where the above option of not doing so does not apply, the problem may arise of obtaining full overbite reduction, or maintaining full reduction once achieved.

General arch levelling may be sufficient to reduce anterior overbite to edge-to-edge, but if it should be insufficient and it has been necessary to engage the archwire in the bicuspid brackets, the component of force from the posterior anchor bends which should continue incisor depression will fall on the brackets of the bicuspids, particularly the second, and will take time to filter through to the anteriors, whilst placing strain on the anchor molars.

In these circumstances the archwires can be given a general curvature in the vertical dimension, as was described in conjunction with second bicuspid extraction cases.

The curvature imparted to the upper archwire conforms with an exaggerated curve of Spee, whilst that for the lower arch represents a reverse curve of Spee. The introduction of these curvatures increases the reciprocal elevation and depression which takes place between the bicuspids and the teeth of the labial segment, whilst reducing the vertical strain on the molar anchorage (*Fig.* 9.10).

Treatment Example *b*

The second hypothetical example to show the mechanics of appliance treatment following first permanent molar extraction is submitted, not to cancel anything which has already been said, but to add to it.

It was assumed in respect of the first treatment example that the teeth of both dental arches were reasonably well aligned and therefore Stage 1 procedures could immediately be inaugurated.

Where overcrowding is more severe it becomes necessary to bring about alignment of the individual units by using auxiliaries, looped archwires and elastic ligatures where indicated. The resulting balance of movement must be clearly foreseen. It must also be seen that the mechanical components associated with the object of general alignment do not interfere with the smooth action of the Class II elastics, i.e. frictional resistance to the free sliding of the archwires. If this should be the case, particularly where anchorage may become critical, it might be advisable to wait general alignment before instituting full Stage 1 mechanics.

Example *b* shows a manifestation of dental overcrowding in the lower arch, in which there is displacement of the buccal teeth *en bloc* in one direction, as opposed to individual misplacement in various directions.

The teeth of the buccal segments, including cuspids, are often found to be forward of their respective labial segments, either in one or both arches. This means that the cuspids occupy a markedly labial position relative to the incisors, with variable amounts of imbrication of the latter. The relationship of the cheek teeth may be Class I in these circumstances.

In example *b* (*Fig.* 9.2*b*) the lower incisors, although imbricated, occupy an acceptable position antero–posteriorly and an acceptable angulation to the mandibular base. The upper incisors are proclined into a position of overjet, producing Class II division 1 incisor relationship.

If a plain or looped lower aligning archwire is fitted the wire will stand well to the labial of the lower incisors in the first instance, because of the position of the lower cuspids. Inevitably, when alignment of the lower labial segment takes place, the crowns of the lower incisors are bound to be moved considerably towards the lower lip, which would create, in this example, a situation resembling bimaxillary protrusion. Subsequently the lower, as well as the upper, labial segments would require retraction until they reached their estimated stable antero–posterior positions. This means that the lower labial segment would have to undergo a 'round trip'. Had the upper labial segment been not proclined, but normally related to the lower, with the cheek teeth in the same positions, the relative prominence of the upper cuspids would have caused the upper incisors ultimately also to have to undergo a 'round trip'.

It could be argued that such 'round trips' are not really necessary and that aligning incisors by first proclining, before subsequently retracting, makes the attaining of a precise target for the eventual position, antero–posteriorly, of the labial segments, difficult and arbitrary.

If there were no other way, the double incisor movement would have to be accepted, but there remains the option of leaving the incisors undisturbed until space has been gained for their alignment by independent retraction of the cheek teeth, including the cuspids. In the current example the option applies to the lower arch, and can be carried out by the following procedure.

Bands and attachments will be fitted to the second molars, cuspids and bicuspids, in a conventional manner. An 0·018 in. archwire is then fitted which, either by conventional means or by a recurved system, gives the required molar control against mesial tilt, mesio–lingual rotation and lingual roll. The main wire is engaged in the cuspid and bicuspid bracket slots, but carried free of the incisors. If the unsupported labial section of the archwire should impinge on the lower lip, it will be necessary to adapt this section by stepping it in towards the incisors, by insert bends placed at the mesial of the prominent cuspids. If an undue intrusive force is delivered to the bicuspids, notably the second, from a recurved pattern of archwire whose main section lies beneath the lower molar buccal tube, a vertical height adjustment bend will have to be incorporated in the main archwire, in the region of the first molar extraction site. In the case where conventional archwire is used, the standard anchor bend being used for molar control, if any height adjustment is required, it will probably be to avoid elevation of the bicuspids, and consequently it will be in the opposite direction to that described above for the case where a recurved system is used. This would also be the case where double archwires and oval tubes are employed.

Independent retraction of the cuspids and bicuspids is motivated, on an intra-maxillary basis, by the application of elastic ligature or chain. In order to reduce frictional resistance in the bracket slots from tooth rotation, the elastics can be applied both to the labial and lingual of the teeth. In the case of the lingual aspect, cleats will be required on each tooth, including the molars, whilst on the buccal the existing brackets will provide support. Little force is required since the teeth to be retracted are permitted to tip, which helps conserve molar anchorage. If doubt or fear exists as to molar anchorage response, the number of teeth retracted at any one time can be reduced.

Whether independent retraction is undertaken in one or both dental arches depends upon the nature of the case and will be at the operator's discretion. Once the cuspids and bicuspids have been retracted, the brackets of the incisors can be engaged and alignment completed, the 'round trip' having been avoided. Stage 1 can then be completed, followed by Stages 2 and 3 in the usual manner.

The presence of lingual cleats will have a further function in Stage 3, after extraction spaces have been closed, notably for those cases for which molar control has been by the use of oval tubes and double archwire. It is not possible in these cases to hold the space closed by bending the distal ends of the archwires round the buccal tubes. Instead, a continuous ligature must be tied to the lingual cleats to produce the same safeguard (*see Fig.* 5.3).

Conclusion

Any reader who would prefer to have been given one simple method for dealing with all situations which might arise from extraction of first permanent molars, may be disappointed by the apparent existence of so many alternatives.

Essentially, what has been prescribed is the standard application of the Begg technique, with the addition of various means for correcting or controlling the roll of the second molars, where needed.

The observation has also been made that, in circumstances of marked labial displacement of cuspids relative to incisors, the application of any form of Stage 1 general alignment archwire would be bound to effect unnecessary labial movement of the incisors, from which position they would later have to be retracted. Separate retraction of the cheek teeth avoids probable detrimental effects which could stem from the double incisor movement, without adding to anchorage cost.

Neither of these additions seriously alters the standard use of the Begg technique as the basis for treatment procedure.

It is not possible to cover every minute permutation of possibility by giving a detailed course of action for each; there are too many. To attempt to do so might appear to simplify, but in reality would be bound to oversimplify, which might cause thought to be withdrawn just when it is most needed.

Asymmetrical Extraction

It happens that patients can present who have already had extractions carried out for reasons other than orthodontic, or possess teeth inviting extraction because of their poor condition, or who have the misfortune to have teeth congenitally absent. Spaces may already exist, or have to be created, in the dental arches which may or may not be so located as to ideally suit the needs of orthodontic treatment. Consideration must be given, nevertheless, to the prospects for orthodontic treatment if use is to be made of existing space or that created by enforced extraction, with respect to the resultant standard and the overall time to be taken. In the most unfavourable situations, it may be necessary to extract further teeth in order to obtain workable space and anchorage advantage. Fortunately such conditions are rare and it is more likely that effective use can be made of the space resulting from enforced extraction and missing teeth, but, because the spaces are seldom ideally located, mechanical procedures may be in some ways atypical.

Certain circumstances could bring about asymmetrical extraction, for example, the removal of a bicuspid from one side of the arch and the first permanent molar from the other. So long as the space created is sufficient for the accommodation of the remaining teeth and for the estimated anchorage requirements, the standard Begg technique can be applied with little alteration.

Where extraction has been asymmetrical, care will have to be taken that appliance mechanics do not subsequently create asymmetries which do not exist in the first place.

If a bicuspid has been extracted from one side

of an arch and the first molar from the other, it is probable that an archwire with anchor bends of identical size on either side will be found, on insertion into the buccal tubes, not to lie parallel to the horizontal plane in the incisor region. The reason is that the archwire is fitted into a second molar tube on one side and a first molar on the other, making for different lengths of archwire on either side. The anchor bends may need to be adjusted so that anteriorly the archwire lies in the horizontal and produces an even intrusive force, both left and right, on the labial segment.

Where the above extractions have been carried out in the lower arch, the use of the second molar one side and the first on the other also produces a discrepancy in the distance between the upper inter-maxillary hooks and those on the lower molars, so that the force produced by the same size elastics is greater one side than the other; but this is not usually detrimental.

It is always likely, in the asymmetrical extraction case, that a feature of treatment in Stage 2, will be the advent of unilateral space closure. The full engagement of the archwire on the side of closure and the use of uprighting springs in a capacity as brakes to arrest unwanted local shifts of teeth has been described earlier as part of the description of the basic Begg technique.

Chapter 10

'Multiple extraction' and non-extraction treatment

In the opinion of most people, the removal of four teeth as part of orthodontic treatment, might well rate as 'multiple extraction'. To the orthodontist, however, the extraction of four units is so commonplace that he reserves this colloquialism to describe those treatments which have involved the removal of a larger number of teeth.

General Considerations

It is now accepted by most that a proportion of occlusions presenting for orthodontic treatment display overcrowding of the teeth to a degree which could never be assimilated by any reasonable expectation of future growth, and consequently the only hope of permanent relief lies in the reduction of the number of teeth by extraction. Usually one unit from each quadrant, four teeth in all, will suffice. In cases where overcrowding is exceptionally severe, the logical question is raised as to whether further extraction is justifiable.

When considering the matter of extraction in general terms it would seem reasonable to assert that the decision upon whether or not to extract, and if so how many teeth, should be a purely diagnostic issue related to the nature of the case, and not to be influenced or dictated by the mechanics of any appliance. The latter may eventually have some influence, through the requirements of anchorage balances, upon where to extract, but not upon whether to extract, nor upon the number of teeth to be involved.

The orthodontic appliance should be an instrument in the hands of the operator, capable of bringing about any tooth movements which he considers both possible and appropriate to the best treatment of the individual. It should not, through any built-in limitation, tell him, in effect, what is appropriate.

Theory of Attritional Dentition

Dr Begg has underwritten a policy of extraction, derived from his study of the skulls of ancient Australian aboriginals, to which he has added an interpretation of his findings to endorse an approach to treatment of modern malocclusion.

He found that the teeth of these skulls showed marked occlusal and interproximal attrition which could be attributed to the eating habits and diet of the aboriginal in primitive times. The wearing down of the incisor teeth, through the early establishment of an edge-to-edge occlusion, to the narrower parts of the teeth, coupled with the same process in the buccal regions and interproximal wear, resulted in the dental arches being shortened by the equivalent of a unit either side, by the time the aboriginal was twenty years of age. Such conditions were conducive to health of the gingival tissues and caries was not prevalent. Dr Begg concluded that the human dentition was designed to meet these primitive conditions by being provided with excess tooth tissue to compensate for gradual loss through wear. From these observations Dr Begg propounds his 'Stone Age Man's Attritional Dentition' theory.

Modern man, unlike his prehistoric ancestors, lives on a soft diet which does not contain even low percentages of sand or other abrasive substances. Attrition is consequently an almost non-existent feature of present day occlusions. The complement of teeth however, has not been altered by the passage of time.

From this it can be argued that if attrition has not claimed a unit of tooth material from the arch length during the patient's first twenty years, it would be correct to obtain the same balance by eliminating that amount by extraction.

Discussion

Full acceptance of the theory would virtually make extraction obligatory in every case where the full dentition has developed. An exception would be provided by some individuals who possess the full complement of teeth which are, nevertheless, spaced. No orthodontist would feel inclined to create yet more space by extraction in such a situation.

One cannot help but be reminded of the theory of non-extraction propounded at the turn of this century by Dr Angle, and the fierce debate he, Dr Case and their respective aides had over the issue. It would now appear that the concept of 'never extract' is being replaced by one of 'always extract'. One of the theories must be wrong—or perhaps both.

If man does indeed possess excess tooth material, and this could be proved to be a fact and not an assumption, could this be a compensation not only for attritional loss, but other forms of loss, such as through caries or periodontal disease, both of which are encouraged by present day diet? Periodontal disease may strike late in the patient's life, but some attention to the possibilities of the future should be given when planning treatment of the occlusion. Part of an orthodontist's concern must be to assist the patient to conserve his dentition and not to help him get rid of their teeth by extraction, unless strictly necessitated by their dental condition.

There are occlusions for which the standard of treatment result and long term stability are undoubtedly improved if associated with extraction. The profile and general facial aesthetics also benefit, in these cases, from the same action. Equally there are occlusions which, if treated by extraction methods, may be stable, but are not so acceptable either from the point of view of the facial profile, or that of the active treatment period, which can become unnecessarily protracted. Both of these detrimental features usually stem from the requirement to close excessive space within the arches, and can still happen even when the principle of reversal of anchorage has been applied.

It would seem that it is not possible to base treatment universally on either extraction or non-extraction. Either way there will always be exceptions. It is true that, if it were possible to lay down a fixed rule, it would mean, amongst other things, that subsequent appliance techniques could be largely standardized and much thought and worry thereby taken from the mind of the orthodontist. It may be that this realization was behind the ideas of both Dr Angle and Dr Begg when their treatment concepts were originally propounded.

In the case of Dr Begg, the standard use of his appliance in three clear cut stages possesses an alluring, albeit deceptive, simplicity, and the allure would be that much the greater if the method could be applied to all treatments more or less regardless of detailed consideration.

The successful operation of the Begg technique demands the existence of space within the dental arches to allow for both tooth alignment and anchorage movements. This is sometimes supplied by nature, but where interproximal contacts exist throughout the arches the space must be created by extraction. Even where tooth alignment is good, any use of Class II elastics will eventually cause forward movement of the entire lower dental arch, unless space has been created to accommodate movement of the posterior anchor units mesially without, at the same time, moving the lower labial segment labially into a position of doubtful natural stability.

It follows that, in cases which have, prior to treatment, gross overcrowding of the arches, the removal of four first bicuspids may yield only enough space for the general alignment of the teeth, with little or no space left to allow for any shift of the anchor units. This means that interproximal contact is reestablished early in the mandibular arch and thenceforward the continued use of Class II elastics would threaten mesial movement of the whole lower dentition, in the same manner as in the non-extraction situation described above. Inadept or careless handling of mandibular anchorage would aid or, in the worst circumstances, actually create the same predicament. One way in which Class II traction could be continued would be by creating more space by instituting further extraction. The case concerned would then become one of 'multiple extraction', justification for which could be obtained from the degree of initial overcrowding, backed by the attritional dentition theory.

There is probably a very small minority of

occlusions which do indeed display massive overcrowding, to a degree that the removal of four units would fail to suffice for alignment, let alone anchorage movements. In these rare instances additional extraction may be necessitated by the nature of the case; but such radical action should not be taken solely to gratify the anchorage demands of the appliance mechanics.

Where first bicuspid extraction provides space enough for general alignment, but some little remains thereafter, the case for additional extraction is less strong, in that the residual space might well be adequate for the successful operation of other appliance techniques which, once the extraction sites have been closed in the lower arch, would cease to call on mandibular anchorage and rely thenceforward on extra-oral anchorage.

Those who find that they can accept with no reservations not only the Begg appliance and technique, but also Dr Begg's supporting arguments in favour of extraction, and, where needed, further extraction, can claim that they have no need for the use of headgear. The avoidance of headgear wearing was one element of early propaganda which aimed to emphasize the apparent simplicity inherent in the Begg technique and had an appeal for some orthodontists who either had a dislike of headgear, or who knew that some of their patients did not cooperate well when asked to wear extra-oral apparatus.

The fact remains that, if intra-oral anchorage has been expended, further anchorage can only be supplied either from extra-oral sources or additional extraction, unless undue shift of the mandibular dentition is accepted. It is a matter for the conscience and judgement of the individual orthodontist as to which method is chosen.

The Begg appliance, by its mode of action, exercises considerable economy in the use of intra-oral anchorage and consequently could be anticipated as having less recourse to headgear than, for example, edgewise appliances; but this is not the same as saying that extra-oral anchorage in conjunction with the Begg appliance should never be considered.

There would seem to be cases who suffer, both as to standard of result and the time taken, if extraction is resorted to in order solely to provide intra-oral anchorage. No appliance system is surely complete unless the option is there to use extra-oral support.

These arguments do not invalidate the Begg technique, still less are they intended to cause personal affront to Dr Begg.

The Begg technique is an efficient means of treating a high proportion of individuals whose occlusions justify the inclusion of extraction and even a rare few whose condition may be so severe that additional or multiple extractions could rationally be contemplated. There are nevertheless borderline cases, some of which would benefit by the avoidance of any extraction, or the avoidance of 'multiple extraction'; and there are also occlusions which would benefit by extraction, but only if carried out in the second molar region. Anchorage support in the majority of such cases would have to come from headgear which, once introduced, would alter the handling of the appliance which could no longer be used in the standard stages of the Begg technique, but which could still be used to great effect through slight modifications to its mode of application. This would widen the already considerable versatility of the Begg appliance whilst not altering the effectiveness of any previous well-tested usage.

Conclusions

The views expressed above have been submitted for consideration in order to try to balance judgement on the vexed question of whether or not to extract as part of orthodontic treatment and can be summarized as follows:

1. Extraction is justified as a means of relieving dental crowding, in circumstances where growth cannot reasonably be expected to provide that relief,

2. The degree of crowding in the average malocclusion of itself rarely justifies the extraction of more than four units. The removal of the four first bicuspids will provide, in most instances, more space than is actually required for tooth alignment, thus allowing latitude for controlled movement of anchor units during appliance treatment;

3. Extraction of more than four units is justifiable in the comparatively rare conditions wherein arch crowding is so gross that the space created by the removal of four first bicuspids only just permits, or is actually inadequate for, the theoretical alignment of the remaining teeth;

4. Supplementary extractions should not be

performed for the sole purpose of providing further expendable intra-oral anchorage in order that Class II mechanics can be continued. The appliance and attendant technique should be modified for some treatments, so that use can be made of extra-oral anchorage in lieu of lower arch anchorage and to avoid over indulgent use of tooth extraction, and

5. The introduction of the possible use of headgear would not invalidate the Begg technique. The use of the Begg appliance in the classic three stages would remain a viable treatment approach, but not the only one.

The foregoing remarks are not intended to dispute the facts concerning the existence of tooth attrition in primitive times, nor that the absence of such wear might contribute in some measure to the manifestation of overcrowding so frequently encountered in present day occlusions. If doubt exists, it is as to whether the attritional dentition theory can really be extended to justify extraction as an almost universal expedient.

Dr Begg has come close to creating a standard three stage system of appliance treatment which could be universally applied to any malocclusion. For the appliance to be used in the recommended manner, space must exist within the dental arches. The required space is not often supplied by nature and therefore must be created artificially by extraction.

It becomes necessary therefore to support the appliance system with a plausible theory which would make space creation by extraction acceptable and thereby to placate the mind of any orthodontist who might be unwilling to remove teeth where the requirement was not obvious, or where in his opinion, the obligation could be avoided if an alternative mechanical system were to be used. If the theory of Stone Age man's attritional dentition has been submitted to this end, one is entitled to speculate as to whether the tail has not wagged the dog, in that the means has promoted the theory rather than the theory justifying the means.

Orthodontic Extraction and the Growth Factor

A plea has been made in the foregoing section to keep the role of extraction strictly in line with the nature of the case. Judgement of the need or otherwise for extraction is usually based on the symptomatic evidence of overcrowding of the dentition, i.e. tooth displacement from the line of the arch and rotation. This method of judgement is the best practical approach, because growth prediction has not yet reached a point of reliable accuracy.

In fact, when the permanent teeth erupt they take up positions dictated by the balance of local environmental factors at that particular point in time. Subsequent growth, in all three dimensions, will have altered that balance before orthodontic treatment is commenced. This does not necessarily mean that the original tooth positions will improve spontaneously, but the growth increase will have improved, to some variable extent, the potential for general tooth alignment by appliance, without recourse to extraction. More growth can be anticipated during the period of active orthodontic treatment, which would further facilitate non-extraction alignment. The question that is raised concerning the treatment of each individual, is whether the total growth increase before and during orthodontic treatment will be sufficient to so alter the environmental balance that the teeth will be tolerated in their new positions, bearing in mind that it will be necessary to increase the dental arch dimensions to overcome crowding by antero—posterior or lateral expansion. Obviously the greater the initial overcrowding, the smaller the chance that average growth would compensate for the degree of expansion which would be needed to attain alignment. If the patient is not to grow to accommodate his dentition, the dentition must be reduced in size to fit the patient; and this means resort to extraction. This is one area where one would wish for a means of accurate growth prediction per individual rather than to have to rely on averages.

The influence that the growth factor can have on treatment results can be studied retrospectively. Case reports are published from time to time, some of which show unusually large amounts of overcrowding having been accommodated by a non-extraction procedure and the result shown to possess good post-retention stability. The object of the publication is often to arouse admiration for the skill of the perpetrator, but, if the opportunity is offered to study the extent and pattern of growth, it will be seen that the operator, skilful though he may be, has been given a favourable wind by the growth factor, which accounts more for the accomplishment. Other cases, which are far less likely to be given the glare of publicity, show some measure of failure of non-extraction treatment to deal with comparatively mild initial overcrowding. Perhaps overbite reduction may not reach the full extent in these cases, or, following the discontinuation of retention, one or more units may pop silently from the line of the arch. Less than average amount of growth in one dimension or another is as likely to be the underlying cause of such apparent failures as any other factor.

Treatment of the Multiple Extraction Case

The contrasting cases described above represent left and right of average in respect of the growth contribution to orthodontic treatment.

It has been conceded that initial overcrowding may be of such monumental proportions in some individuals that more than four units might need to be removed, which leads to the necessity of describing the technical handling of such treatment.

The Timing of Extractions

Before embarking upon that description, one further issue of importance must be mentioned. This concerns the timing of the extractions and the effect on the duration of active appliance therapy.

It can happen that gross incipient crowding of the dental arches is seen early by a general dental practitioner who perhaps finds, at the same time, that the first permanent molars are poorly calcified, carious or have been extensively restored. The combined circumstances may cause him to advise the removal of these teeth on the grounds that the space created will permit the remaining teeth to become less entangled during the eruptive period, so that the orthodontist will be later faced with a simplified problem. The degree to which this policy succeeds depends on a number of factors. Unfortunately, sometimes there is little or no sorting out of those teeth anterior to the extraction sites, and the main natural tooth movement which takes place is the mesial migration of the second permanent molars. By the time the orthodontist is called upon, the second molars may well have moved bodily forward two-thirds of the first molar extraction space, with little mesial tilt. The remaining third of the extraction space could prove

inadequate for the accommodation of the grossly crowded anterior segments, let alone allow for any anchorage movements. If additional space is to be obtained, the orthodontist is faced with two possible alternatives. He must either attempt to move the second molars distally, or indulge in further extraction.

Bodily distal movement of the second molars of both arches over any appreciable distance would be a time consuming task requiring headgear. Even if space is regained, there is the possibility, where apical positioning is unfavourable, that it cannot be used without the bodily retraction of the bicuspids, making a long treatment even longer.

It can come about in this way that the second alternative is preferred and the first bicuspids removed. The case has now become one of 'multiple extraction'. Working in conjunction with slight excess of space is undoubtedly less time consuming than treating in the presence of inadequacy. It is easier to close space than to fight for its recovery, although this fact should not necessarily endorse extraction or additional extraction.

The space created by the removal of the first bicuspids will be taken up by the alignment of the grossly imbricated teeth. The residual third of the first permanent molar extraction sites will provide intra-oral anchorage for the use of intra- and inter-maxillary elastic forces as the second molars are moved mesially into contact with the second bicuspids.

Treatment in the above circumstances should be no more difficult, nor time consuming, than the treatment of the ordinary first bicuspid extraction case and result should be of high standard. In view of the early loss of the first permanent molars, it is to be hoped that the third molars have developed so that the patient has the expectation of a reasonable complement of molar teeth.

The situation becomes very difficult if no early intervention has taken place and the crowded dentition has been allowed to develop intact. Because of the degree of crowding, some teeth may have been unable to erupt and of those that have, many can be expected to be considerably out of alignment. If the marked crowding is judged to be so severe that the extraction of eight teeth is justified, the choice will fall on the first bicuspids and the first permanent molars. This choice permits the use of reciprocal intra-oral anchorage and, once space closure has taken place, the second bicuspid will intervene between the cuspid and the second molar, making for a better appearance of the end result than if molars contact the cuspids.

With the removal of the eight units at the same time an immense amount of space is created. The archwires will be relatively long, with little support in the buccal regions, particularly if the second bicuspids have been unable to erupt to schedule. The archwires for Stage 1 alignment and overbite reduction would be in consequence potentially vulnerable to damage, and the lower one may need to be stepped gingivally to avoid interference from the cusps of upper bicuspids, if erupted.

Much of the extraction space will eventually be taken up as the displaced units are brought into the arch by the usual Stage 1 procedures, but this may take longer than usual because of the severity of the original malocclusion and the probability of having to wait upon the eruption of some of the teeth.

Even after general alignment has been achieved, it will still be necessary in Stage 2 to close some two thirds of the original first molar extraction spaces. Where this procedure involves the lower molars, much time will be required for its completion. This will be true even if the lower second molars have not rolled lingually, nor tended to do so during treatment and so require correction.

These are amongst the reasons why, when eight units are extracted from grossly crowded but nevertheless intact arches, at or near the same point in time, the subsequent appliance treatment often extends to two and a half or even three years' duration. This is in complete contrast to the eight unit extraction case which happens to have come about by stages through the early removal of the first permanent molars as previously described. In the latter instance the overall treatment period need not exceed that for the standard first bicuspid extraction case.

In the above contrasting examples it is the distance the second molars, notably the lowers, have had to be moved mesially which has had the greatest influence on treatment time; yet if the distance is reduced by dint of early extraction of the first molars, the action is accompanied by a measure of uncertainty. For example, will the third molars develop? How much will the patient grow? How much natural improvement will take place? Will the final mechanical intercession be timed correctly, or will the patient find him or herself far from orthodontic assistance when the time comes? These are the type of question which may not be easily answered when considering planned early intervention.

In some cases, the dictates of circumstances will confine the need for supplementary extraction to the upper dental arch. The closing of the upper first molar extraction space by the mesial movement of the second is neither particularly time consuming nor difficult; it is the same movement for the lower arch which is associated with these disadvantages.

Appliance Technique for Multiple Extraction Treatments

When multiple extraction is undertaken, the teeth removed are usually the first bicuspids and first permanent molars in preference to eight bicuspids, in order that a more pleasing balance is set at the conclusion of treatment. It is as well to know, before removal of molar teeth, that the third molars are present by checking their size and position by radiograph. It is to be hoped that, when the second molars are to be moved to take the place of the first, the third molars can erupt to take the place of the second. If third molars happen to be absent or have to be removed, the course of treatment might have to be based on the use of extra-oral rather than on reciprocal intra-oral anchorage, which would represent another occasion for the possible use of headgear with the Begg appliance, and involve different mechanical procedures to those described below.

Stages

The mechanical stages for the eight-tooth extraction case, are set out in *Figs.* 10.1, 10.2 and 10.3, in the context of Class II division 1 with associated gross overcrowding.

The treatment procedures are an amalgamation of the techniques for the first bicuspid extraction case and the first permanent molar extraction case. The similarities to the conventional Stages 1, 2 and 3 can be seen. The objectives of each stage will be as usual and as follows:

For Stage 1:
1. To obtain general alignment of the individual teeth of both arches;
2. To reduce overbite and overjet; whilst
3. Correcting the molar relationship.

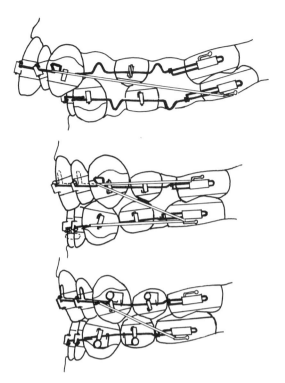

Figs. 10.1, 10.2 and 10.3. Stages 1, 2 and 3 of the treatment of a multiple extraction case with removal of first permanent molars and first bicuspids.

These objectives should all be reached before introducing the Stage 2 space closing procedures involving the use of the customary complex of inter and intra-maxillary elastics.

In Stage 2, if the space to be closed is so great that the threat exists of over-retracting or 'dishing in' the anteriors, the tendency should be countered by the application of distal root movement auxiliaries to the cuspids and/or anterior torque spurs for palatal or lingual root movement of the incisors.

When judging whether the labial segments are threatened with over-retraction, the reaction of the dental arches as a whole to the Stage 3 root movement auxiliaries should be borne in mind. It is probable that these will create a general forward shift of both arches and therefore the labial segments should be somewhat over-retracted at the end of Stage 2 by way of compensation. Over-retraction beyond this point should be avoided.

Stage 3. When all spacing has been closed, the Stage 3 objectives will be, as usual, to parallel and reposition those roots that were, or have become, displaced.

The auxiliaries which can be used for the purpose have already been described. Which of these are used, and where, depends on the exact nature of the situation at the completion of Stage 2 and will vary a little in accordance with the pattern of the original occlusion. In the case illustrated, for example, the upper bicuspids have a distal inclination and will require root correction in the opposite direction to that which is typical in a first bicuspid extraction case. The orthodontist must assess the sum of all anchorage effects inclusive of any such anomaly.

Molar Tubes

As a result of general alignment, the space created by the extraction of the first bicuspids will probably be used up and some of the first molar space encroached upon, but whatever the demand for the use of the molar space, it is difficult to claim more than a third by the bodily retraction of those teeth anterior to the gaps. The residual molar space will perforce have to be closed by the mesial movement of the second molars. The amount of space to be closed in this way will vary, but will often be considerable.

The situation therefore will demand the same mechanical control against mesial tilt and lingual roll over the second permanent molars as they are moved mesially as was described for the first molar extraction case. Indeed, once alignment and space closure has been brought about in the anterior segments the remainder of treatment becomes essentially the same as for a first molar extraction case.

The options on the use of oval buccal tubes and a redoubled archwire, or round buccal tubes used with plain or recurved archwires, can be used in accordance with the observations and instructions contained in Chapter 8.

Archwires

The fact that an occlusion has warranted the removal of six or eight permanent teeth implies the presence of much crowding and consequent tooth displacement. The early Stage 1 archwires should therefore be of light gauge for alignment of the labial segments, but, in view of the long spans, probably unsupported and unprotected in the buccal regions, flexibility through the use of loops will often be more appropriate to the scene than flexibility gained through small gauge archwires. In order to provide resistance to possible damage and to provide adequate depression force to the anteriors from modest sized anchor bends, 0·018 in archwires are preferred as soon as practical to 0·016 in. If, through the absence of teeth, or the presence of only partially erupted teeth, in the buccal segments, the long spans of archwire between the cuspids and the second molars appear to be exceptionally vulnerable to potential distortion from masticatory forces, the archwires should be stepped gingivally. This is no more than the customary rule for the circumstances and refers to archwires with no bracket support in the buccal regions. Once bracket engagement is contemplated the fitting sections must be restored to their proper relative heights.

Where gross crowding of the dental arches is present, one common effect is a marked displacement of the cuspids labially. If this state exists and ideal alignment archwires are fitted, the incisors will be moved labially, the cuspids being more resistant to reciprocal distal movement because of their larger root area. If the incisors become unnecessarily proclined in this matter, it will become obligatory to retract them to their proper position of balance at some later stage. Stage 2 of treatment provides the opportunity in theory and, so long as the labial displacement of the incisor teeth during alignment has been of modest proportions, in practice as well. On the other hand, where alignment has caused one labial segment or the other, or both, to become excessively tilted towards the lips, there may be grounds for concern as to whether full recovery can be accomplished before the available anchorage is expended. The thought is also promoted that it is probably poor policy to move a labial segment far in one direction for little more than the amusement of getting it back again if there is any way by which this can be avoided.

As mentioned in an earlier context, the above problems can be resolved if the labially displaced cuspids are retracted separately by intra-maxillary elastic from cuspid lock pin to the buccal hook on the molar. Since only simple tipping of these teeth is sought, the elastic force need be no more than 30 g. The main archwire is left free of the incisor teeth or, if support in that region is thought necessary, so adjusted as to fit passively in the central incisor brackets. It is unlikely, in a multiple extraction case, that there will be any shortage of molar anchorage, particularly in the lower arch. Use of separate cuspid retraction in the above manner is most applicable to the lower arch, where the final position of the labial segment has so much influence on the natural stability of the entire treatment result. One would not wish to jeopardize the critical positioning of this segment by moving it any further away from its original position of equilibrium than can be avoided.

The archwires will carry the usual inter-maxillary traction hooks or rings and anchor bends. If a redoubled archwire is used in oval tubes, the double section is wound on to the main archwire at the point where the anchor bend is placed. As usual, looped archwires will be replaced by plain ones as soon as the bracket alignment permits. Class II elastics are worn continuously.

One further feature of the Stage 1 and 2 archwires which can be seen in the diagrams is the presence of vertical loops opposite the extraction sites. These can be incorporated to shorten the archwire and so keep the anchor bends in their proper relationship to the molar tubes as the large amount of excess space is closed. By so doing the number of new archwires needed over a period is reduced.

It should be emphasized that these loops should not be contracted whilst the archwire is in position in the mouth. Their closure would adversely affect the degree of posterior anchor bend and reciprocal anterior overbite control, but, with the archwire in situ, these effects might not be apparent.

As in the first permanent molar extraction case, at the point where bicuspids are fully engaged with the archwire, interference to the anterior depression force to control or reduce overbite can occur through the bicuspid absorbing most of the anterior component of force from the anchor bend. Rather than increase the posterior anchor bend, a general curvature is imparted to the archwires in the vertical dimension, representing, in the upper arch, an increased curve of Spee and, in the lower, the corresponding reverse curvature.

Stage 3 archwires, components, purpose and mode of application for the multiple extraction case do not differ from those described thus far for other forms of treatment.

Conclusion

Much of the technique for dealing with the multiple extraction case is the same as that given in previous contexts. In order to avoid too much repetition, attention has been concentrated on those issues which are particularly relevant to treatment by multiple extraction. It is hoped that the reader will be able to fill in the rest of the picture from what has gone before in this text. He should have least difficulty if he has concentrated on the reason why this or that action is taken and not tried to form set mental patterns for archwires or any other features. It is the principles behind the patterns that matter.

The Treatment of the Non-Extraction Case

The Begg technique, when first introduced, appeared to be essentially an extraction based form of treatment. The appearance was created by the practical necessity of having surplus space available within the dental arches in order to allow for the movement of anchor units during treatment. In most instances this space can only be introduced through extraction. The impression of an extraction technique was further enhanced by the appended theory of the 'attritional dentition', which seemed to be aimed at endorsing the respectability of the extraction approach. In consequence there were those who were surprised and impressed by the first reports of successful treatments accomplished using the Begg technique without extraction.

The majority of these early case reports on non-extraction treatments, when examined critically, did not give rise to wonder at their success. If there was a mystery involved, it was not that extraction had been avoided, but that such a measure, by implication, had ever been seriously considered. Extraction had been avoided because the dental arches, far from being crowded, actually displayed natural spacing so situated and of such dimensions that compensation was afforded for the anticipated anchorage shifts. A fortuitous situation existed which made the provision of space by extraction as unnecessary as it was undesirable.

Further reports have since been submitted, the success of which is less obvious to explain, in that little or no natural spacing existed prior to treatment and no use was made during treatment of headgear to supply anchorage. Usually these cases are of the minor discrepancy type, wherein there are no extensive overjets or individual tooth displacements. The absence of overcrowding in successful non-extraction treatments is to be expected, but is a factor insufficient to explain all. One or other, or all, the following additional factors may be present in order that final success can be achieved:

1. Growth since the eruption of the first permanent molars and incisors may have been sufficient to permit modest degrees of arch expansion to be incorporated in the treatment plan. Such expansion may be either antero—posterior or lateral or both. This, together with continued growth during active treatment, alters the volumetric environment three-dimensionally, so that new positions for the teeth can become both possible and stable;

2. Lower arch anchorage may have been greater than usual, through the control given by the cortical plates to the lower incisors against tilting. If the lower incisors happen to be housed within a narrow isthmus of supporting bone, the amount of labial tilting which might result from a general mesial movement of the lower arch in response to the application of Class II elastics is limited, which effectively helps to increase the lower arch anchorage potential; or

3. Use may have been made of mechanical measures, e.g. lower labial root torque auxiliary, for the reinforcement of lower arch anchorage.

Lower Arch Anchorage

Unless some use is made of extra-oral anchorage, it follows that the required anchorage must be found from intra-oral sources. The standard Begg technique depends for its operation upon intra-oral anchorage and, in particular, that provided by the lower arch or, in association with space, sections of it. So long as space exists in the lower arch, either naturally or by extraction, a section of the lower arch can be used to supply anchorage and the resultant shift accommodated without disturbing the teeth of other segments.

In the non-extraction case where inter-proximal contacts exist throughout the lower dental arch, any forward movement of the molars in response to Class II elastics will be transmitted to the arch as a unit, gradually causing the lower incisors to tilt labially, unless restrained by factors described in either items 2, or 3 above. This labial movement of the lower incisors, and the amount to which it takes place, can be used as a measure of lower arch anchorage expenditure. The question is immediately raised as to how much labial movement of the lower labial segment can be tolerated and at what point such movement comes to represent an unacceptable anchorage loss. This matter has already been argued at some length earlier in this book and there is no need to repeat the theories and systems of assessment previously mentioned. They will be just as relevant to the non-extraction case as for those involving extraction, or, as some may think, just as irrelevant. The amount of labial displacement of the lower anteriors which will be tolerated, without subsequent imbrication, cannot be accurately quantified by any known simple method, such as reference to the APo line. Even if an accurate system of assessment were to exist, it is unlikely that the precise latitude for labial movement of the lower anteriors would be necessarily the same for any two consecutive cases.

It comes about that there are those who consider the safest policy is to leave the position of the lower labial segment as little disturbed antero—posteriorly during treatment as possible, making only occasional exceptions. Others, working to theories suited to their own beliefs, help themselves to considerable latitude when determining the final position of the lower labial segment. Whatever may be the personal convictions of individual orthodontists on the vexed question of the conditions governing the ultimate stability of the lower dental arch, it is still necessary to describe the amount of anchorage which can be expected from an intact lower arch and the measures which can be taken to produce the maximum possible resistance.

In a non-extraction case wherein the lower arch displays good alignment with full interproximal contact throughout, the application of Begg brackets and a plain Stage 1 archwire will allow tipping to take place for all but the first molar teeth. The latter, through the presence of the anchor bends, alone have any measure of bodily control. The resistance of the lower arch to mesial movement from Class II elastics will be little more than the minimum, unless an increased resistance of the lower incisors, through the medium of the cortical plates, happens to exist. If such control is absent, even the lightest inter-maxillary force will soon be liable to cause mesial movement of the

entire lower arch. If this shift is to be kept within reason, both the force application and its duration must be kept to a minimum. Fifty grammes over a period of six months might well prove near the limit, if instability of the lower incisors is not to be introduced. It might also be mentioned that, if heavier forces are employed, the lower arch may stand up well initially, giving rise to false confidence that it will continue to do so indefinitely. Confidence evaporates when a seemingly sudden and unacceptable mesial shift of the lower dentition takes place, as a result of accompanying undermining bone resorbtion.

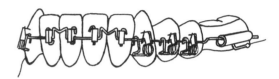

Fig. 10.4. A means of obtaining maximum mandibular anchorage by use of mildly active root paralleling springs and torque archwire, which collectively produce a braking effect by bodily control against forward displacement from the inter-maxillary elastic pull.

It stands to reason that if the maximum resistance is to be obtained from the lower arch, full bodily control should be mechanically provided to each tooth, or better, actual apical leverage supplied to them in a mesial or labial direction.

In the case of the Begg appliance, the above arrangement can be achieved by applying labial root torque to the lower incisors through spurs bent into the main archwire or by the fitting of an auxiliary (*Figs.* 5.10 and 5.11). In addition, mesial root movement auxiliaries can be fitted to the cuspids and bicuspids. Initially these springs should be mildly active. As soon as there is mesial movement of the dentition through the application of Class II elastics, the springs will become more active, so acting as brakes. The total arrangement is illustrated in *Fig.* 10.4.

The overall mechanical effect is similar to that which would be obtained from an edgewise set-up, with appropriate brackets, rectangular wire with labial incisor root torque and second order bends (tip back) in the buccal regions. Indeed, from the point of view of convenience and oral hygiene, the lower edgewise appliance would be a deal less clumsy and every bit as effective.

One would not wish, however, to encourage the mixing of techniques, particularly where the use of the Begg appliance is concerned. The temptation to do so often exists and may be yielded to in the hope of obtaining the best of both worlds, but where coordinated and correlated tooth movements are being carried out (which is the usual situation) the Begg appliance should be used in both arches, if full advantage of the system is to be obtained. The mixing of techniques is unprofitable in the main but, where the objective in the lower arch is not movement but the supply of anchorage, as in the above situation, there would be nothing lost by the use of an edgewise appliance for that arch.

Whatever means of bodily control used, no more can be hoped for than that lower arch resistance has been brought to a maximum against the effect of Class II mechanics. This still does not ensure that the lower arch cannot be moved. Movement in a mesial direction will occur if the arch is overexposed to the traction force. Due to the bodily nature of the tooth movement, anchorage loss may be less clinically obvious than when tilting has been permitted, and regular monitoring of the relative position of the lower labial segment by lateral skull radiographs will be needed.

Lower arch anchorage is therefore both precarious and limited. It is also variable from individual to individual and difficult to quantify prior to use. Consequently the extent of the tooth movements which can be safely carried out, using the lower arch as anchorage, is also limited. Matters are only changed if space exists in the lower arch to permit segmental anchorage movements without disturbing the arch as a whole.

Extra-Oral Anchorage

It is seldom easy to work on the shifting sands of intra-oral anchorage and, where the use of an intact lower arch for anchorage purposes is concerned, clinical judgement and appliance mechanics are perhaps at their most critical. Any slight error in either can lead to a situation where the faults in the original occlusion become gradually exchanged for new faults which were never there in the first place.

Consequently most orthodontists seek greater anchorage security in the circumstances. If this cannot be introduced through space by extraction, or should not be, the only other alternative is to cease to call upon the lower arch and turn to the use of headgear.

Headgear forces can be applied either to a Kloehn type bow fitted into second buccal tubes

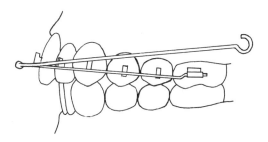

Fig. 10.5. Lateral view of Kloehn type facebow placed in the occlusal of the two buccal tubes and stopped against the tubes by bayonet bend to maintain the anterior of the bow clear of the incisor teeth.

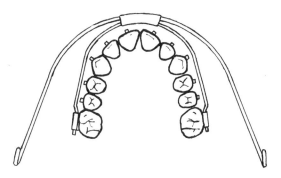

Fig. 10.6. Occlusal view of Kloehn bow. Stops to maintain the bow free of the anterior teeth are provided by bayonet bends against the buccal tubes. The same bends permit clearance of the brackets on the buccal teeth.

placed occlusally to that containing the intra-oral archwire on the upper anchor molars (*Figs.* 10.5 and 10.6), or direct to the anterior of the archwire. In the latter case, the upper archwire is provided with additional rings bent in mesial to the upper lateral incisors, into which the hooks on the headgear arms can be latched, *Fig.* 8.6. (*Figure 10.7 illustrates two designs of straight and high pull headgear.*)

If some space exists in the upper arch and it is desired to continue retraction of the upper labial segment, the headgear force is applied to the anterior of the arch, the mesial migration of the molars being prevented by conventional anchor bends.

Once space has been closed, but further distalization of the arch as a whole is required, the extra-oral force can still be applied to the anterior of the archwire. It is appropriate in these circumstances to place molar stops in the main archwire in contact with the molar tubes, so that arch length is maintained.

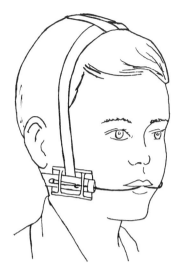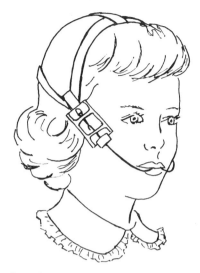

Fig. 10.7. Straight and high-pull headgear. Many alternative headgear designs are available, including those for combined straight and high pull and for variable force direction.

If the aim is not to move the upper arch distally, but to control it against mesial shift in response, for example, to palatal root torque of the anteriors and/or distal root movement of buccal teeth, the same stopped archwire and anterior application of the headgear arms is still viable.

The alternative approach for either distal movement of the upper arch, or the stabilization of the upper arch against forces tending to displace it mesially, is to apply the headgear force by Kloehn bow to double tubes on the molars. If and when this is done, it should be realized that, however the arms of the bow are adjusted, there will be a tendency for the anchor molars to tilt distally, which will reciprocally cause the anterior of the archwire to descend occlusally, with detrimental effect on anterior overbite. It might be thought that the incorporation of conventional anchor bends would offset this latter effect. In fact, the anchor bends assist the bow to tilt the molars distally. With the one force augmenting the other, the amount of molar tilt can soon become wholly undesirable. The amount of anchor bend should not exceed that which is needed to cross the lumen of the tube. Some control over extrusion of the anteriors can be gained by incorporating an increased curve of Spee into the main archwire, but the threat of excess molar tilt still remains from the extra-oral bow itself.

Since it is difficult to eliminate the distal tilt of upper molars when the headgear forces are applied to them, many make it a rule that, if extra-oral anchorage is to be used at all with the Begg appliance, the force should always be applied to the front of the arch. In this latter use watch must be kept for molar expansion resulting from compression of the archwire anteriorly.

Headgear forces of around 250 g should be sufficient for the purposes described. The free tilt form of the brackets should be borne in mind and spacing amongst the upper anteriors, if present, eliminated and thereafter kept closed by mutual ligation during retraction.

Appliance Mechanics for the Non-Extraction Case

The basic mechanics for the non-extraction case can perhaps best be described in association with a mild Class II division 1 occlusion which happens to possess some natural spacing within each dental arch. The existence of the spaces provides a certain latitude for controlled anchorage movements. The latitude may, or may not, be sufficient to accommodate the anchorage response to the whole tooth movement programme, but, even if it did not, it would be difficult to justify extraction in any occlusion which exhibited spacing prior to treatment. Therefore the best use must be made of the available anchorage. If the point is reached where it is judged that continued application of Class II elastics would cause undesirable mesial shift of the lower arch following the closure of the space, the remaining tooth movements must then be carried out with headgear support.

Treatment can be initiated, and probably completed, making use of the space available and the standard three-stage Begg technique. Stage 2 of the conventional approach will almost certainly be eliminated, since it is unlikely that available space will be in excess of requirements.

Bands and brackets are placed on the first permanent molars, incisors and cuspids of both dental arches. There is no need to band the bicuspids at this stage, unless any require the correction of rotation. Overbite and overjet reduction will be facilitated if the bicuspids are left unbanded.

The main archwires will be equipped with the usual inter-maxillary hooks or rings placed mesial to the cuspid brackets. In addition, where some or all the bicuspids are unbanded, loop stops some 3 mm in height are incorporated sufficiently to the mesial of the buccal tubes to allow spacing to close, but not to overclose. In other words, they are there to preserve arch length and prevent the continued use of inter-maxillary traction from squeezing the unattached bicuspids out of line. The stops do not interfere with the conventional anchor bends which will be placed mesial to the loops. When the archwires are fitted, the inter-maxillary hooks are ligated to the wire immediately distal to the cuspid brackets.

The Stage 1 archwires are made of 0·018 in gauge wire partly because of greater potential resistance to damage to the long unsupported buccal spans and partly to minimize the size of the anchor bend angle suited to the provision of an appropriate force for overbite reduction. A further safeguard against damage to the buccal spans of the lower archwire from the cusps of the upper teeth can be provided by stepping the archwire gingivally in the area between molars and cuspids. These steps need be only mild to achieve their purpose and, once space in the dental arch has become closed, the distal step can be allowed to contact the anterior of the buccal tube and thus act in the same way as a loop stop in preserving arch length.

In view of the probably precarious nature of the anchorage, the inter-maxillary force should be kept as light as possible, supplying around 50 to 60 g. *Figures* 10.8 and 10.9 show the appliance arrangements described above.

If any of the bicuspids happen to require correction, it follows that the offending teeth will

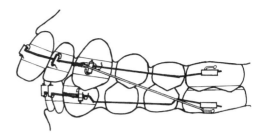

Fig. 10.8. Non-extraction. Reciprocal closure of space in both arches resulting in the elimination of mild overjet. Loop stops can be placed in both archwires sufficiently to the mesial of the molar tubes to allow space closure, but not to permit overclosure when the bicuspids are not engaged with the archwire.

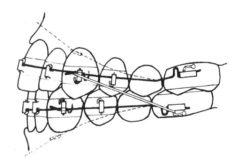

Fig. 10.9. Where, for any reason, it has been necessary to engage bicuspid brackets, the main archwire may need to be curved, as shown by the broken lines, in order to complete overbite reduction, or hold previous reduction. The use of posterior anchor bends alone, in this circumstance, overstrains molar anchorage causing them to tilt distally.

also have to be banded. If the displacements are either in the vertical or bucco–lingual directions, correction will be through the main archwires, with or without incorporated vertical loops. If rotation correction is needed, loops or elastic ligatures are employed. It will probably be appropriate to most non-extraction cases if the correction of bicuspids is left till the latter part of Stage 1, because loops or elastic ligatures are apt to interfere with the free sliding of archwires, obstructing both overjet reductions and lower arch anchorage movements. Once the bicuspids are banded and engaged with the archwire, here, as elsewhere, one effect is to reduce the effectiveness of the posterior anchor bends to either maintain, or assist, overbite reduction. An increased curve of Spee should be introduced into the upper arch and a reverse curve into the lower, whilst actually lessening the usual degree of the molar anchor bends themselves.

Stage 3 will involve correction of apical displacements using the usual auxiliaries deployed to suit the requirements of the case. It is unlikely in most non-extraction cases that extensive amounts of root movement will be needed, which in turn will reduce the demand on the critical anchorage resources.

The supply of lower arch anchorage may prove to be equal to the demand, or may run out at some point during treatment. No more can be done than to use all mechanical means of giving bodily support to the units of the lower arch and to keep Class II traction forces light. If, after that, the threat of lower arch displacement arises, either extraction has to be belatedly performed, or the remainder of the treatment programme completed with extra-oral anchorage support. Many orthodontists, when faced with cases offering borderline decisions respecting the need to extract, commence treatment on non-extraction lines and observe results carefully. They find this 'therapeutic diganostic' approach helpful in coming to a final conclusion as to whether or not to institute the irreversible act of extraction.

Chapter 11

Synopsis of factors influencing the pattern of the adult occlusion

The foregoing text has concentrated primarily on the problems of Class II division 1 occlusions and the mechanical means, through the Begg appliance, for the correction of the associated malrelationships of the teeth. By so doing the majority of the components of the appliance and their purpose have been described. It remains to show how these same components are deployed for the correction of Class II division 2, Class III and Class I occlusions and to demonstrate any modifications to the basic Begg technique which might consequently be necessitated.

Although the main purpose of this book remains the description of the mechanics and technique for the use of the Begg appliance, it is difficult when discussing the use of any appliance, to stand entirely aloof from the causative elements of the various forms of occlusion which are to be treated. Nowhere is this more the case than when dealing with the treatment of Class II division 2. Results of treatment of this type of occlusion, through Begg or any other appliance system, tend to vary from the highly acceptable to those perhaps best described as disappointing. The reason for the variable nature of treatment results lies in the variability of the supporting and surrounding structures and their relationships rather than of the teeth themselves, or of appliance mechanics. This statement would be true of the treatment of other forms of occlusion; but the possible anatomical limitations which can be met in Class II division 2 are perhaps less immediately obvious.

Because the underlying causes of Class II division 2 are still something of a mystery to some, it could be worthwhile, with research material available, first to present a summary of general factors concerned with the eventual pattern of the occlusion, followed by a detailed comparison between the development of Class I and that of Class II division 2, with particular reference to the variables involved in the latter. By so doing, it is hoped that the judgement of the relative prognosis of proposed Class II division 2 treatments can be improved and the appliance mechanics involved rationalized. At the same time, attention will be focused on the effects of the interplay of variables, as an example of the way in which differing occlusal patterns can be produced.

General Aetiology of Occlusal Patterns

The eventual pattern of the adult occlusion results from the influence of human variation as it pertains to the teeth and elements of their immediate environment in each individual. For an occlusion to develop which is both aesthetic and functionally satisfactory, variation within the above elements must be limited and proportionately balanced.

So long as variation is slight, there is the possibility of natural compensation through small adjustments in the form or position of the dento–alveolar structures. Where this does not take place, or where variation is more marked, orthodontic measures will have to be taken to bring about the desired end mechanically. Orthodontic treatment will have varied success, depending upon the extent of the original variations and growth potentials.

In cases exhibiting extremes of variation of the facial components, the balance of the occlusion may be so adversely affected that orthodontic measures alone cannot provide an acceptable result, in which circumstances surgical intervention may have to be called upon to assist or provide the solution.

The Influence of Elements of Dental Environment

The following is a brief description of the manner by which the elements, broadly indicated above, influence the pattern of the adult occlusion.

The Facial Skeleton

If the adult occlusion is to develop so as to be acceptable from all dental standpoints without orthodontic treatment, the shape, size and relationship of the maxilla and mandible must be coordinated. Individuals in whom there is a lack of such coordination will have varying potential for buccal crossbites, overjets or reverse overjets.

Mandibular size and shape also influence, in conjunction with its controlling musculature, the amount of inter-maxillary space the dento–alveolar structures have to cross during their vertical development, both anteriorly and posteriorly. Marked increase of the anterior vertical height of the lower face, usually associated with a high gonial angle, can result in the combined vertical growth potential of the upper and lower dento–alveolar structures proving inadequate to cross the increased space, producing an anterior open bite.

The opposite situation of small anterior lower face height, often with an associated low gonial angle, does not necessarily induce deep incisor overbite, although probably increasing the potential to that feature.

The general pattern of the facial skeleton is established early and, by the time orthodontic treatment is contemplated, little further change in relationships is to be expected as growth continues. The basal skeleton imparts a three dimensional influence on the shape, size and relationship of the dental arches. The alveolar ridges, both in cross sectional form and relationship, are further influenced by the pattern of surrounding soft tissues within which they develop.

The Oral Soft Tissues

The alveolar structures, containing initially the deciduous teeth, develop vertically on their bony foundations to cross the inter-maxillary space and have to do so within the confines of the lips and cheeks on their buccal aspects and the tongue on the opposite side.

Since these soft tissues are connected to the main skeleton, variation in the latter may be reflected in the former, resulting in slightly different relationships in the individual between the lips and the incisor teeth and the cheeks and the buccal teeth. In addition, the soft tissues themselves are subject to morphological variation from individual to individual, independent of the underlying skeleton.

The cross-sectional shape of the developing alveolar process is modified through bone deposition being inhibited in areas permanently, or semi-permanently, occupied by the soft tissues. In this way the bone becomes moulded to a form convenient to the freedom of muscular action and, by the same means, the summit of the ridges become established in an area of comparative quiescence within muscular activity.

The pattern of the alveolar ridges thus established influences the path of eruption of the permanent teeth by guiding them through the peripheral shape of the bone towards the crest of the ridge where they will eventually erupt in positions unobstructive to normal oral function, unless prevented by the presence of supernumerary teeth, some element of pathology, accidental damage or congenital defect.

As soon as the crowns of the permanent teeth break surface and enter the oral cavity, they come under the direct influence of the local musculature. Their positions will be modified by the forces falling on them, so avoiding any obstruction to the ease of muscular function which might otherwise have been promoted.

The crowns of the teeth will eventually take up position of equilibrium in most instances and in others of near equilibrium. In the latter instance their own bulk and mutual support has altered the equation.

In some individuals the lower lip may be of such a pattern as to restrict the extent of the bone support bucco–lingually for the lower incisors to such a degree that these teeth are prevented, by the narrowness of their support, from tipping labially on eruption in the usual manner in response to the demands made by the tongue action. The lower incisors are not always, in these circumstances, in a position suited to ease of function of the tongue, which has to adapt to the situation in speech and swallowing, particularly in the presence of lip incompetence. In milder cases, the lower incisors are merely restrained to a more vertical position which can either add to the size of the overjet, or permit the upper incisors to retrocline as in Class II division 2 occlusions. The retroclination of the upper incisors is one way by which natural compensation can be given to eliminate a potential overjet, the other being the proclination of the lower incisors. In cases where the bony isthmus containing the lower incisors is narrow, the latter form of compensation is automatically limited.

The amount of inter-occlusal clearance between the teeth or either arch with the muscles at rest (freeway space) would appear to be determined by the masticatory forces delivered to the crowns during function; but the vertical growth potential of the alveolar processes, particularly the lower, may well have a considerable influence. There are those individuals, often with Class II division 2 occlusions, who have alveolar heights which are substantially below average, but who also display above average inter-occlusal clearance with the muscles at rest. When the teeth are brought into occlusion there appears in these cases to be an overclosure of the mandible with some forward rotation at the condyle.

Further examples of the influence of the soft tissues on the occlusal pattern are to be found in the description of the overbite factors and in the account of the development of Class II division 2 given elsewhere in this text.

The Teeth

The size and number of the permanent teeth should be balanced with the accommodation afforded by the supporting bone. Failure of such accord will produce either overcrowding of the dentition or spacing of the individual units.

The presence of supplementary teeth may interfere with the eruption of others or contribute to arch crowding, just as a congenital absence of teeth may increase spacing.

Teeth of unusual form or crown root angle may contribute to malalignment of the dental arches or interfere with their proper occlusion.

Failure to erupt most commonly affects the cuspids, notably the uppers, and is probably due to the inability of the buccal or lingual cortical plates to give proper guidance to teeth whose developmental angle fails by a large margin to coordinate with the guide planes. Some teeth develop horizontally within the bone, often upper cuspids; but the phenomenon is occasionally seen elsewhere amongst other units.

Pathology, Trauma and Habits

Damage to the facial structures, inclusive of the teeth, through accident or disease, must necessarily have an effect on the occlusion, not least if it should occur during the period of development. It is not possible in this form of brief survey to summarize the permutations of cause and effect which could arise out of the above statement, nor to enter into the problems created by the congenital disaster of cleft palate and the related effects on occlusal development. Conditions arising out of these factors must be treated on merit with a view to producing the best possible result in the adverse circumstances.

As to habits, that most commonly met by the orthodontist is finger- or thumb-sucking. The presence of either can, over the period of tooth eruption, cause the displacement of the incisor teeth and sometimes distortion of the anterior alveolar processes. The effects are usually as short lived as the habit itself and, if not actually self correcting, can be eliminated by orthodontic treatment at the appropriate time. The cause may be psychological, but sometimes appears to be partly physiological, in that the patient may find that the process of swallowing is facilitated in his case by the intrusion of the thumb which assists the provision of an anterior oral seal, more usually supplied by the lips. It is no coincidence therefore that most patients with the thumb-sucking habit also have a Class II division 1 malocclusion with Skeletal II relationship of the apical bases, together with an inability to approximate the lips, either as a result of deficient lip tissue, or through the adverse pattern of the facial skeleton, or both. The malocclusion would have existed without thumb-sucking. The latter has been induced and may, or may not, aggravate the occlusion still further.

The same may be said of another way in which swallowing can be facilitated, namely by the use of the tongue against the inner suface of the lower lip to promote anterior oral seal. The same type of cases are involved and the nature of the tongue action, helps to maintain the overjet and incomplete overbite.

In most instances thumb-sucking is voluntarily discontinued when orthodontic treatment is instituted, if not earlier; but the use of the tongue against the lower lip may persist as an aid to the function of swallowing even at the conclusion of orthodontic treatment, and become a factor in relapse.

Study of the Eruptive Behaviour of the Permanent Incisors

Through a study of the eruption of the incisor teeth, from development to full eruption, an interesting indication can be gained of the manner in which the permanent teeth respond to their immediate environment by alterations of long axes angles and relative positions, so contributing to the eventual pattern of the developed occlusion. These small but significant changes are additional to any malrelationship of the dental arches brought about through aberrations of the facial skeleton.

The records of 42 patients (11 Class I, 16 Class II division 1, 8 Class II division 2 and 7 Class III) who had had annual lateral head radiographs taken between 4 and 12 years of age, were examined by the author, for the purpose of finding out whether there was any pattern of incisor eruption which was sufficiently consistent within all groups of occlusions that it could be described as typical. If this should prove to be the case, the next intentions were to discover the range of variation within the sample as a whole and for sub-groups and, if possible, to supply logical reasons for the movements and the variations. Observation was not centred on the movement of the incisor tips alone but also on the open apices, so that a picture could be built up of the behaviour of the tooth as a unit during two periods, the first whilst still immersed in bone and the second from the moment of eruption until that process was complete.

The comparatively small size of the sample and uneven distribution of the numbers representing the Angle occlusal classifications, were both due to the scarcity of patients who had been regularly radiographed from as early an age as 4 years. The nature of the sample had to be borne in mind when drawing conclusions.

During the pre-eruptive phase, whilst the developing central incisors were within the alveolar bone, it was found that 57 per cent of upper centrals became more perpendicular to base as their tips approached the summit of the ridge; the same process affected 60 per cent of lower centrals. The opposite movement occurred in 29 per cent of upper centrals and 13 per cent of lowers, the remaining cases showing no alteration in long axis angle. The range of long axis change, during this period, was from an increase of 12° to a decrease of 13° for the upper centrals and from an increase of 11° to a decrease of 17° for the lowers.

These changes, when viewed as an average for the sample as a whole, showed that the incisal tips of the upper and lower centrals moved slightly labially whilst their apices moved rather more in the same direction, resulting in a few degrees decrease in long axis angle relative to base. There was little actual difference shown, during this pre-eruptive period, between one class of occlusion and another.

Closer inspection revealed the probability that the incisors of either arch were guided by the peripheral shape and angle to base of the investing bone, towards the point of eruption near the summit of the ridge. Whether the centrals proclined or retroclined during their passage towards final eruption depended therefore on the initial development angle of the teeth relative to that of the alveolar process; the pattern of the latter had long since been established during its initial development and the eruption of the deciduous teeth.

The alveolar pattern, to which the teeth respond, remains comparatively unchanged in most individuals from 3 years of age onwards, unless orthodontic treatment is instituted. Alteration to shape, as opposed to an increase in size, does occur without artificial aid in a small minority. Another temporary phenomenon, affecting a minority, is a gradual bucco–lingual enlargement of the upper alveolar process to combat the situation where the process, at this time, is relatively small but the contained incisors large. Where this 'pregnant' situation develops tooth eruption is invariably delayed.

Once the central incisors began to emerge into the oral cavity, the positions and angulations became directly influenced by the presence and activity of the surrounding soft tissues, with the result that more positive changes were observed.

The lower centrals increased their long axis angle in 97 per cent of the sample, only 3 per cent showing very small amounts of the opposite trend. The maximum increase for any individual was 28°, whilst the maximum decrease only 2°. The average expectation was for an increase of 11° in the angle between the lower central and the mandibular plane during this period up to full eruption.

The upper incisors showed a more variable behaviour than the lowers. The upper central incisor long axis increased to base in 56 per cent of cases, whilst the opposite occurred in 36 per cent, with 8 per cent showing no change. The maximum individual increase was 19° and the maximum decrease 24°. It would not surprise anyone to learn that the maximum increase was related to a Class II division 1 occlusion and the maximum decrease to division 2.

Table 11.1. **Maximum change in angle SNI found in any one arch**

	Before eruption		After eruption	
	Angle increase	Angle decrease	Angle increase	Angle decrease
Upper central	7°	2°	8°	2°
Lower central	4°	2°	10°	2°

Table 11.2. **Maximum change in angle SNI over full eruptive period in any one patient and average change for full group**

	Maximum change		Average
	Angle increase	Angle decrease	Angle increase for group
Upper central	13°	1°	5·2°
Lower central	11°	1°	5·2°

Because the balance of the various Angle categories within the sample used in this study would not be representative of the community at large, the percentages given would only be true of this specific sample.

It should also be observed that description of tooth movement by reference to changes in long axis angle alone can be misleading. For example, if it is said of a given individual that the lower centrals proclined 10° after eruption and the uppers retroclined 10°, an impression is created that the crowns of the lowers have moved considerably to the labial whilst those of the uppers have moved palatally. It is difficult to avoid mentally equipping the teeth with hinges fixed at some point on the roots. In fact the behaviour of the erupting incisors resembles more than that of an object immersed in fluid than one with any fixed form of attachment. Crown and apex can move in the same direction, but the one more than the other resulting in a long axis change as well as a general movement. In addition to the angular changes of the central incisors to their maxillary or mandibular bases, it was therefore necessary to fix the positions of the incisal tips relative to the Naison at each stage throughout the eruptive period. For this purpose the angle SN to incisal tip was used.

During their eruption through bone, the tips of the upper centrals moved labially in 68 per cent of the sample and the tips of the lower centrals moved labially in 55 per cent. No change in the angle SNI was recorded for 26 per cent of upper centrals and 29 per cent of lowers. Palatal movement of the upper incisal edge was confined to 6 per cent of the sample and lingual movement of the lowers to 16 per cent.

During eruption into the oral cavity, labial crown movement took place in 82 per cent of upper centrals and 94 per cent of lowers. Lingual or palatal crown movement was found in 9 per cent of uppers and 3 per cent of lowers, the remainder showing no change. As can be seen in Table 11.2, where lingual or palatal movement of the incisor edges was encountered, the amount of movement was very small.

When the changes in the angle SNI are taken into account together with the long axes changes, the contribution made to the latter by the movement of the apex can be assessed.

The Development of Class I Occlusion Contrasted with that of Class II Division 2: The Eruptive Behaviour of the Upper and Lower Central Incisors in the Two Types of Occlusion

In order to give specific example of the events described in general terms in the previous part of this chapter, the development of Class I incisor relationship has been chosen to illustrate the eruptive behaviour of central incisors when within a well balanced skeletal framework and soft tissue environment.

Alongside Class I development, and for the purpose of direct contrast, the events taking place at comparable movements in the production of Class II division 2 incisor relationships have been described and illustrated. *Figure* 11.1 shows the two classes of occlusion at 4, 6 and 12 years of age. The middle age group conveniently coincides with the upper central incisors reaching the point of eruption.

Although the diagrams have been greatly simplified so as to leave only the bare essentials, the shape, size and relationships of the structures shown are not the product of imagination. The original diagrams were geometrically constructed from the averages of 85 coordinated measurements taken from each of the serial lateral skull radiographs of 8 Class I and the same number of Class II division 2 occlusions. The measurements enabled the relative positions of 32 points on the facial skeleton, including the incisors and their supporting bone, to be established so that, using the averages for the two groups, an accurate graphic representation could be built for each chosen stage of development. The SN line was used as base for the geometrical reconstruction. In addition to the skeletal morphology and tooth position, both deciduous and permanent, one soft tissue landmark, namely the summit of the red margin of the lower lip, is indicated by the point of intersection of the lines seen in the diagrams labial to the incisor teeth. The long axis angle of the incisors, whilst still only partly calcified, was assessed through the use of templates constructed to the form of the central incisors as seen when fully developed in the later radiographs. The template was superimposed on that section of the tooth which had so far calcified when the radiographs of the patient, when younger, were taken.

The Class I sequence demonstrates what can be regarded as the typical eruptive behaviour of the central incisors. From their earliest measurable position, the permanent upper and lower central incisors become, on average, a few degrees nearer perpendicular to the maxillary plane as they proceed towards the point of eruption. The incisal edges move labially, but the open apices move slightly more in the same direction, resulting in the angular change.

On eruption, the lower incisors tip labially under the influence of the tongue, almost invariably with movement of their apices towards the lingual. The upper central incisors also tip labially on eruption, usually with some accompanying shift of the apices palatally. The tipping movements which occur at this time are the same in character as those brought about by simple spring forces from appliances. The movement is completed by full eruption, after which the tooth positions become relatively stable.

The contrasting Class II division 2 sequence shows little difference of practical significance to Class I at either 4 or 6 years of age in the matter of permanent incisor eruptive behaviour, except the expected difference in general skeletal pattern. Once erupted, the lower incisors tip labially as did those of Class I; but, on average, to a slightly lesser degree in Class II division 2. The average figure, as is so often the case, conceals the truth. The labial tilt of the lower incisors is not consistent case by case, but shows considerable variation. Some cases involved in the Class II division 2 sample possessed a lower anterior alveolar process which was much narrowed bucco–lingually due to a particular pattern of lower lip which intruded into the area where bone would otherwise have been deposited on the buccal aspect of the process. The narrowing of the bony section which results effectively controls the amount of labial tilt of the contained incisors possible by movement at either crown or apex. Indeed, the isthmus of bone containing the lower incisors can be reduced to a width no greater than the tooth roots, in which case there may be no change in tooth angle on eruption.

The upper central incisors of Class II division 2 do not tip labially on emerging from bone as did those of Class I, but tip in the opposite direction, often to a marked degree. Most of the tipping is brought about by labial shift of the incisor apices, the pivotal point being near the necks of the teeth. The tilting is terminated either by prevention by the buccal cortical plate of any further labial apical shift, or, more frequently, by the crowns of the upper centrals reaching the obstruction of the tips of the lowers.

The upper incisor retroclination is caused by the presence of the lower lip as the teeth erupt within its cover, so long as they do not encounter obstruction from either the lower incisors or other teeth of the upper arch. Although it will be found that the lower lip to upper incisor overlap is an average of 6 mm in Class I division 2 and 3 mm in Class I occlusion, the amount of overlap is only one issue in the production of division 2 incisor relationships. The remaining factors have still be to described.

The Formation and Establishment of a Class II Division 2 Incisor Relationship

The preceding study of serial average diagrams of developing Class I and Class II division 2 occlusions

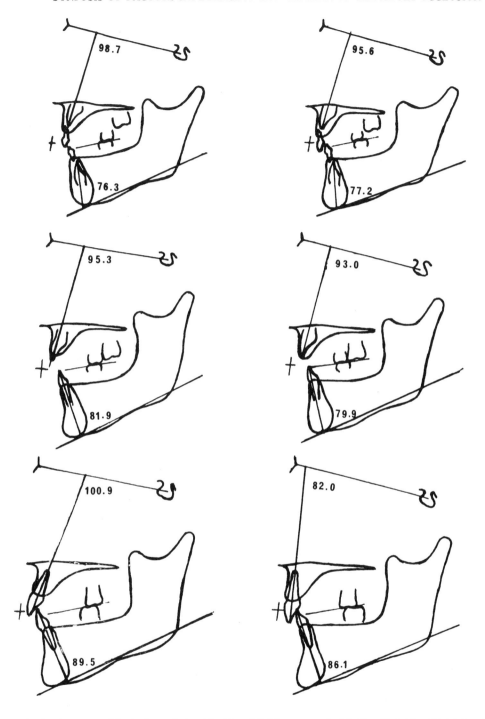

Fig. 11.1. The development of the incisor relationship. Class I (*left*) contrasted with Class II division 2 (*right*) at 4 (*top*), 6 (*middle*) and 12 (*bottom*) years of age. The diagrams have been constructed from averages, derived from the facial dimensions taken from serial radiographs of eight young developing patients in each occlusal category. [4 years: I, SNIU 76·3°, SNIL 73·7°; II 2, SNIU 76°, SNIL 71°. 6 years: I, SNIU 79·2°, SNIL 77·7°; II 2, SNIU 76·7°, SNIL 72·5°. 12 years: I, SNIU 82·8°, SNIL 80·6°; II 2, SNIU 78·7°, SNIL 76·0°.]

shows that, following eruption, the upper central incisors in the two classes of occlusion behave in a quite contrary manner, the one showing a small amount of proclination, the other a marked amount of retroclination.

In the case of Class II division 2, it can be seen (*Fig.* 11.1) that the upper centrals reach the point of eruption at an angle near perpendicular to the maxillary base, which is no more than a reflection of the fact that the upper alveolar process is similarly vertically placed. The upper incisor long axis angle at this point is nevertheless little different to that of the average Class I case, which has also been induced through the alveolar angle and pattern.

Most of the upper central incisor retroclination occurring in division 2 is brought about during the period between the moment the teeth break surface to the point of full eruption. In some individuals the lateral incisors also react in the same way, but not in others.

For upper incisor retroclination to take place at all, certain preconditioning factors must be present. These concern the shape, size and relationship of facial and dental structures as they relate to the patient's vertical, horizontal and lateral dimensions.

Factors Related to the Vertical Dimension

Amongst the issues of importance to the formation of a Class II division 2 occlusion which arise from the morphologies and relationships of structures pertaining to the vertical dimension, is the motivating cause; i.e. the factor which induces some or all the upper incisor teeth to take up retroclined positions. The point and angle at which the upper centrals erupt must be such that their continued passage towards full eruption takes them inside the fold of the lower lip to an extent that the muco—buccal fold acts as a guide plane producing the tilting movement as eruption continues. The crowns of the centrals may move slightly in a palatal direction, but the root apices invariably move labially to a greater extent, the pivotal point being near the necks of the teeth. The tilting sometimes continues for a period after full eruption, the pivoting occurring around the tips of the lower incisors, which, with a deep overbite, contact at the necks of the upper centrals. When the motive force is exhausted, or the apices of the upper centrals reach the buccal cortical plate, or their crowns the lower incisor edges, the process of retroclination ceases. For the full retroclining effect to be produced the overlap between the tips of the upper centrals and the most superior point on the red margin of the lower lip, measured vertically when the teeth are in occlusion, should be not less than 4 mm. The average found for this dimension in division 2 when the incisors had fully erupted (*Fig.* 11.2) was 6 mm.

Analysis of the serial radiographs of the developing Class II division 2 occlusions did not reveal any clear indication that the lower lip ever delivered more than a mild force on the upper incisors. For example, there was no evidence of the lower incisors being moved lingually after the uppers had contacted them, which might have been expected if the lip force had been high.

It is true that the Class II division 2 patient presents a 'crushed in' appearance, but this is produced progressively, first by the moulding effect of the particular soft tissue morphology on the developing alveolar processes. The effect could be broadly described as a restraining influence, maintaining the processes in an upright position on base, compared with other forms of occlusion. In the second place, the 'crushed' appearance is enhanced by the effect of the lower lip in guiding the upper centrals and sometimes lateral incisors into a position of retroclination.

The large lower lip to upper central incisor overlap is brought about through proportional variations in the vertical heights of the upper dento—alveolar process, the lower lip and the lower anterior facial dimension.

From the measurements obtained from a random sample of 30 14-year-old patients, equally divided as to sex, with Class II division 2 occlusions, diagrams have been produced to show the difference between the third of the full sample which had the smaller lower anterior facial heights and the third which possessed the greater for the same dimensions.

The same diagrams have been superimposed on the average facial form, derived in the same way and at the same age, from a sample of 60 Class I occlusions (*Fig.* 11.3).

The mandibular position in all examples, is that which existed when the posterior teeth were in occlusion.

The position of the superior margin of the lower lip is shown by the cross seen to the labial of the incisors. The most superior point being at the intersection of the two lines.

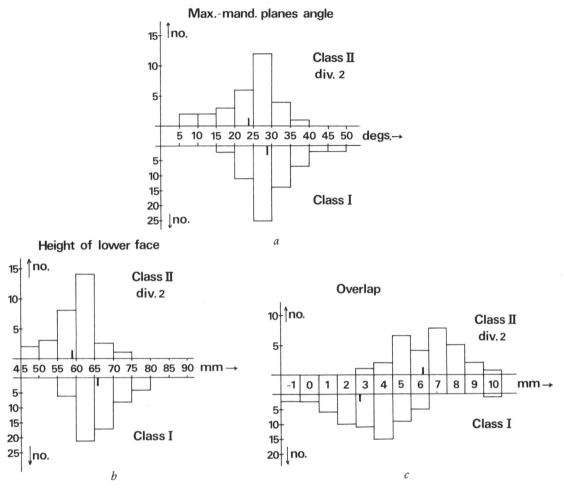

Fig. 11.2. Histograms showing the distribution of three selected features, *a*, the maxillo–mandibular planes angle, *b*, the lower facial height and *c*, the overlap of lower lip and upper central incisor, Class I (a sample of 60) being contrasted with Class II division 2 (sample of 30).

It can be seen from the diagrams of the two Class II division 2 groups (*Fig.* 11.4) that, whether the lower anterior facial height is high or low, the overlap between the lower lip and the upper central incisors still remains, on average, round the 6 mm mark. Clearly, if the proportional balance is similar in each instance, there must be an actual difference in the size of the dento–alveolar structures measured vertically and the height of the lower lip in the two groups. The question arises as to how, in each group, the important lip overlap is achieved, and what the differences are.

In the case of the high lower facial height group of Class II division 2, superimposition on the outlines of the average Class I sample shows that mandibular size and position are almost identical, except in the immediate vicinity of the lower incisors, which appear relatively retracted in the division 2 group. The lower anterior facial heights and the vertical dimensions of the upper and lower dento–alveolar structures are likewise almost identical, on average, for Class I and the division 2 groups. (*Fig.* 11.3.)

The lip to upper central incisor overlap was achieved in some individuals from this division 2 group by the possession of an upper dento–alveolar structure which was proportionately high in relation to the surrounding structures, in some few instances exceeding the Class I average.

More commonly, it was the lower lip which

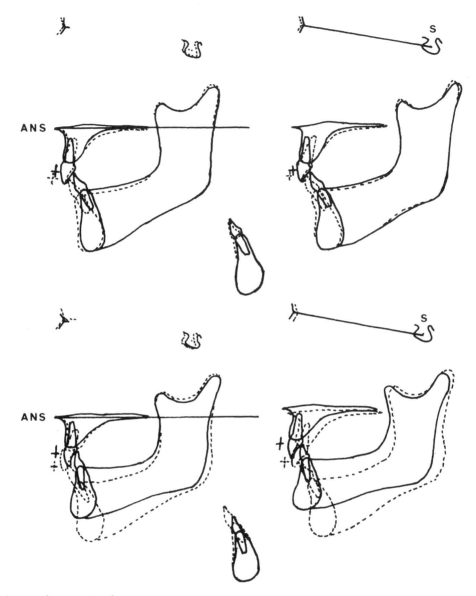

Fig. 11.3. A random sample of 30 untreated Class II division 2 occlusions at 14 years of age was divided into three groups of ten, on the basis of the actual height anteriorly of the lower face. The upper diagrams are superimpositions at ANS and S of the average facial form of the group with the greater face heights upon the product of averages for a full Class I sample of 60 at 14 years of age (dotted lines). The lower diagrams show the average facial form of the 10 Class II division 2 patients with reduced lower face heights, superimposed in the same way on the same Class I outline. (The third group displays a facial form intermediate between the extremes illustrated.)

possessed the increased height, the average being 2·5 mm greater than that for Class I, when measured from the lower border of the mandibular symphysis to the most superior point on the red margin. The effect was produced less by an excess of lip tissue than by the fact that the lower lip, above the fold, was held more erect, or less everted, than found in most Class I occlusions. When contraction occurs during facial expression the lower lip becomes even more erect than when the muscles are at rest. (The lip morphology typical of this type of Class II division 2 patient is shown in *Fig.* 11.8).

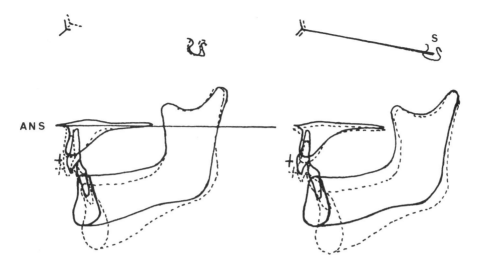

Fig. 11.4. The increased and reduced lower face height groups of Class II division 2 compared by superimposition with each other. This shows group variation. Extremes of individual variation would be that much the greater.

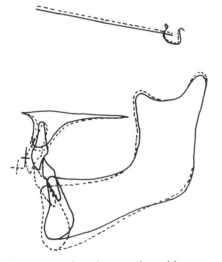

Fig. 11.5. Comparison by superimposition at anterior nasal spine and along the maxillary plane of the average facial form and dimensions and incisor relationships for Class I and Class II division 2 occlusions at 14 years of age. Samples were 60 Class I and 30 Class II division 2 equally divided as to sex. Solid outline represents Class II division 2. Summit of the lower lip is shown by the cross to the labial of the incisors.

In addition to promoting the required lip to upper incisor overlap, this particular lip morphology has a restricting effect on the lower incisors and their bone support, assisting the conditions needed for the formation of a Class II division 2 occlusion in the horizontal dimension as well as the vertical.

In Class II division 2 occlusions with the greater lower anterior facial heights therefore, either the upper dento–alveolar process or the lower lip must attain a height which is increased relative to the rest of the associated structures.

On the other hand, the Class II division 2 occlusions with reduced lower anterior face heights, never possess upper or lower dento–alveolar structures, or lower lips, which exceed the average for Class I occlusions, in respect to the vertical dimension; on the contrary they are invariably well below that average. (*Fig.* 11.3.)

Examining the group of ten Class II division 2 cases, selected from the main sample of thirty as having the smaller lower anterior facial heights, it was found that the average height of the upper dento–alveolar process was 2·5 mm less than that for Class I, whilst the lower dento–alveolar process averaged 5 mm less than Class I, with a lower lip height similarly reduced.

The appearance of the low facial height Class II division 2 group, can be assessed by the superimposition of their average outlines on that of either the high facial height group with the same form of occlusion (*Fig.* 11.4) or on the average outlines of Class I (*Fig.* 11.3). An outstanding feature of the contrasts shown is the posture and position of the mandible on full closure in the low facial height group. There is a lack of alveolar height, not only anteriorly but also posteriorly, causing an appearance of overclosure when the posterior teeth are brought into occlusion, with a forward swing of the mandible at the condyle. This would be natural to the individual concerned and would be tolerated, showing up only by comparison with other groups.

Theories have been put forward in explanation of this phenomenon, but have proved difficult to substantiate scientifically. Broadly speaking, the lack of height to the dento—alveolar structures has been attributed to the strong limiting effect of the occlusal forces which result from the relatively short masticatory muscles, in association with mandibles which have reduced or square gonial angles.

If there exists a low gonial angle, the inter-maxillary space which the dento—alveolar structures have to cross would be reduced, unless compensation was made through the height of the ascending ramus. If the latter was itself less than average, the inter-maxillary space would be less than average even if the gonial angle were not reduced. It is almost axiomatic that the low facial height group of Class II division 2 exhibited individually one or the other of these features, principally the acute gonial angle. Nevertheless, mandibular closure was found to be $3°$ to $4°$ greater than would be expected in the anatomical circumstances.

It was also interesting to note that, where evidence was available, the same patients exhibited an enlarged inter-occlusal clearance, or freeway space, when the muscles were at rest. If, therefore, the overclosure is the result of excess occlusal forces limiting the eruption of the cheek teeth to an unusual degree, why was it that when a bite plate was introduced to relieve those forces, little or no continued vertical growth of the alveolar processes posteriorly took place in many cases of this type? Why, when fixed appliances were used actively to apply elevating forces to the posterior teeth of these same individuals, did the teeth show little response before becoming unusually mobile? Response to these same measures is quite different outside this minority.

Without wishing to add to already existing conjecture, it might reasonably be wondered whether there might not exist at least one further factor. It would seem fair to assume that the occlusal forces are the final limiting factor in determining the height of the dento—alveolar processes posteriorly. In the usual circumstances, when these forces are relieved by the use of an anterior bite platform in cooperative patients, further vertical growth takes place in the buccal regions through release of the residual potential. One result of this is the reduction of anterior overbite. (*See* overbite reduction, p. 66.) In the cases under discussion, the above reaction is minimal or absent, seeming to indicate that there is little or no residual potential to further vertical alveolar growth.

In this minority group, it may be that the lower dento—alveolar structure grows vertically to reach a maximum genetically determined height, albeit one much reduced against the population average. The upper dento—alveolar structure, which appears to be more adaptable than the lower, then attempts to compensate for the lack of height of the lower; but the additional height required to avoid overclosure may exceed the potential of the upper also. Overclosure is then unavoidable and failure to respond when occlusal forces are relieved would also be explained.

From a practical point of view, the facts outweigh the theory. Whatever the true explanation of mandibular size and position, the fact remains that, in occlusion, the lower lip of these individuals, although small by the standard of general averages, is carried high to the labial surface of the upper incisors. The lips, although being of less than average vertical height, have plentiful tissue which is exhibited in thickness. When fully closed, the lips pout outwards and inwards with some overlapping upper to lower. (The typical appearance is shown in *Fig.* 11.8.) This lip pattern is just as effective in guiding the upper incisors into retroclined positions as that described as associated with the high facial height group. Upper incisor retroclination, however, does not necessarily occur simply because the lower lip overlap is great. Other factors must be present before retroclination can take place.

Factors Related to the Horizontal Dimension

Figure 11.6a shows the average dimensions and general form for the ten patients selected from the main sample of thirty 14-year-old Class II division 2 occlusions, as having the least upper incisor retroclination. In direct contrast, *Fig.* 11.6b shows the facial form of those ten patients selected from the same sample as having the most upper incisor retroclination.

One obvious difference demonstrated by this

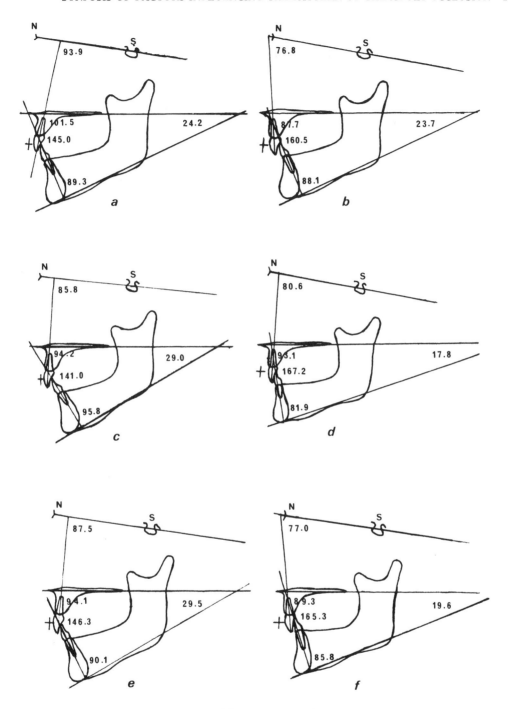

Fig. 11.6. Each of the six diagrams were constructed from the average facial dimensions for groups of 10 individuals, selected from the main random sample of 30 Class II division 2 patients. Selection to each group was on the basis of the contrasting dental characteristics shown against the paired diagrams.

a, Minimum retroclination of upper incisors. Overbite 6·4 mm. *b*, Maximum retroclination of upper incisors. Overbite 7·8 mm. *c*, Minimum retroclination of lower incisors. Overbite 6·5 mm. *d*, Maximum retroclination of lower incisors. Overbite 8·2 mm. *e*, Minimum size overbites (4·8 mm). *f*, Maximum size overbites (10 mm).

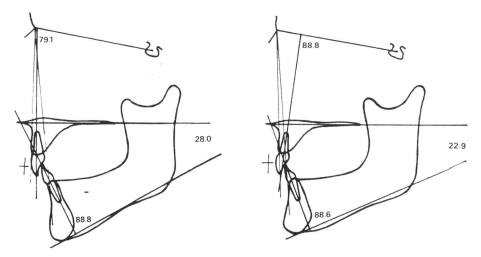

Fig. 11.7. The contrast between the average facial form of the ten cases from the full 14-year-old sample of Class II division 2 having the greatest SNA–SNB angles difference (*left*) and those having the least (*right*). [*Left*: av. SNA 81·2°; av. SNB 73·2° (av. difference 8°); overbite 7·3 mm. *Right* (same data): 78·4°; 75·4° (3°); 6·6 mm.]

comparison is the more marked Skeletal II pattern possessed by the group with the greater degree of upper central incisor retroclination.

This same relationship between skeletal pattern and upper central incisor position can be demonstrated further by selecting from the main sample the ten cases with at least antero–posterior skeletal discrepancy and the ten with the most, on the basis of a greater or lesser SNA and SNB angles difference.

Figure 11.7 contrasts the facial form of those with the greater SNA–SNB difference and with those with the least. It can be seen that upper central incisor retroclination is far greater in the group with the greater skeletal discrepancy.

From the above comparisons it could be deduced that the presence of a Skeletal II pattern is helpful to the production of Class II division 2 incisor relationship, and that the greater the arch discrepancy the greater the anticipated degree of upper central incisor retroclination. If the discrepancy is so great as to be above the critical amount, the erupting upper centrals could be expected to fall onto or outside the lower lip, resulting in a Class II division 1 occlusal relationship.

Although it is a fact that the average Class II division 2 occlusion is associated with a mild degree of Skeletal II patterning, it is probably easier to understand this particular form of occlusion by considering the antero–posterior incisor relationship at the time of eruption. The

presence of a Skeletal II pattern is but one way by which an antero–posterior gap can be created between the already established position of the tips of the lower incisors and that of the upper centrals which have just broken surface.

The upper centrals will continue to retrocline until contact is made with the tips of the lowers, at which point the process ceases if the point of contact is occlusal to the necks of the uppers. This point of contact will vary with the position of the lower incisor tips in both the horizontal and vertical dimensions. Variation will be dependent on the amount of incisor overbite, the mandibular morphology and the angulation to base of the lower incisors and their supporting bone.

In order to investigate the role of the angle of the lower incisors in providing more or less space antero–posteriorly into which the upper incisors can retrocline, the sample of 14-year-old untreated Class II division 2 patients was again used. *Fig.* 11.6c is the facial outline derived from reconstruction of the average dimension for the ten cases selected as having the most labial inclination of the lower incisors. *Fig.* 11.6d shows the outline, obtained in the same manner, from the average dimensions of the ten cases having the least labial inclination of the lower incisors (maximum retroclination). The comparison shows the considerable range of lower incisor angulation, even on the basis of group averages, to be found within Class II division 2. The other obvious difference between the

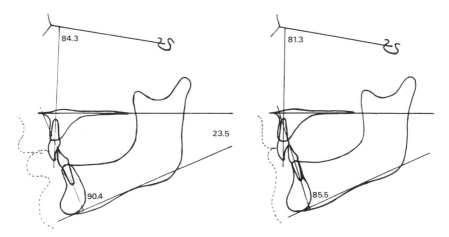

Fig. 11.8. The contrast between the ten **Class II** division 2 cases with (*left*) the wider lower alveolar process opposite point B (av. 9 mm) and those (*right*) with a narrow one (av. 6 mm). The broken outline shows the two types of lip morphology which can be found in association with Class II division 2.

[*Left*: av. SNA 80·8°; av. SNB 74·9° (av. differences 5·9°); overbite 7·4 mm. *Right* (same data): 80·6°; 74·8° (5·8°); 8·3 mm.]

groups, this time not by deliberate selection, concerns the size of the maxillo–mandibular angles.

It was found that, when selecting the ten cases with the least labial inclination of the lower incisors, nine out of the ten cases with the lowest gonial angles were included and the tenth only missed inclusion by 2°. It seemed that the lower the gonial angle, the more upright the whole of the symphysial complex, inclusive of the lower lip. The trend is strong, although not true of all individuals.

The group selected on the grounds of the most labial inclination of the lower incisors showed an almost equally strong tendency to be associated with the higher gonial angles.

In addition to the skeletal influence on the lower incisor and lip positions, the morphology of the lips themselves and their activities, also play a part.

It was stated earlier that, broadly speaking, a Class II division 2 occlusion could be associated with either a lip pattern which was thin and erect, or one which was thick and everted. Not infrequently it was the thin erect type of lower lip which had the effect of inhibiting bone deposition on the labial of the lower alveolar process, thereby restricting the width of the process bucco–lingually, in turn limiting the labial tilt of the lower incisors through control of the cortical plates. The thick

everted form of the lower lip is most usually found in patients with a reduced lower face height and an associated lack of alveolar height. The effect of the thick lip, through its own bulk, is to hold back the lower incisors and their bone support on the mandibular base, providing an appearance of prominence to the mental process. The antero–posterior width of the process is not neccessarily reduced. *Figure* 11.8 shows both, on the right, the ten cases selected from the main sample as having the least width to the lower alveolar process opposite point B and, on the left, those who possessed the most. The characteristic moulding of the symphysial area is to be seen in both diagrams and, in the case of that of the narrow alveolar processes, the effect that this has had in minimizing the labial tilt of the lower incisors is seen.

An example of the way by which mandibular shape and posture in occlusion can combine with locally produced effects on the lower incisor position and angle is provided by *Fig.* 11.9. Here the average pattern of the ten cases with the greatest SNA–SNB angles difference has been superimposed on the average pattern of those ten cases with the least. In spite of the skeletal difference, the tips of the lower incisors have been induced to take up almost identical positions relative to the eruptive site of the tips of the upper centrals.

Many another example could be given of the

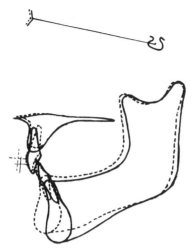

Fig. 11.9. The greater and lesser SNA–SNB angles difference groups superimposed at Sella, showing the similar positions of the lower incisor edges relative to the upper central.

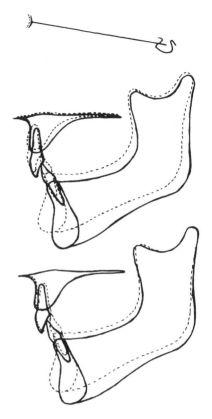

Fig. 11.10. The greater SNA–SNB angles difference group (10 cases) superimposed on the group (10 cases) with the narrow lower alveolar process (*Fig.* 11.8) (broken lines). Shows location of the lower incisor edges, relative to the upper centrals when posterior teeth are in occlusion.

way by which mild maxillary protrusion or mandibular retrusion, assisted by variations of size and posture of the mandible and location and angle of the lower dento–alveolar structure, can combine to produce the required gap between the upper and lower incisor tips at the time of eruption (*Fig.* 11.10). The elements combine in differing proportions per individual, but the effect is the same and, when allied to a suitably large lower lip to upper central incisor overlap, the requirements for the establishment of a Class II division 2 occlusion have almost been met, but not quite. The remaining factor is supplied through variations in the lateral dimension.

Factors Related to the Lateral Dimension

In order to establish the classic Class II division 2 upper incisor formation, wherein the upper central incisors are inclined palatally with the laterals inclined labially, no obstruction must exist which prevents the centrals from becoming thus retroclined. That the upper centrals can be arrested by early contact with the tips of the lower incisors, before becoming clinically retroclined, is implied in the observations above on the horizontal factors; but there is another form of obstruction which is no less effective. This factor is the mutual buttressing of the upper centrals by the upper laterals, which are in turn supported on their distal aspects by the cuspids. For the centrals to retro-

cline there must be no such mutual support, which means that, at the important time of eruption, there must be spacing amongst the upper incisors, or, alternatively, they must be so arranged that the centrals are left unsupported on their palatal aspects.

In order to produce the condition wherein all four upper incisors can become retroclined there must be adequate upper intercuspid width and consequently space to permit the occurrence. Study of the factors in the lateral dimension, therefore, involves:

1. The relative widths of the intercuspid region of the upper dental arch;
2. The relative sizes of the upper incisor teeth; and
3. The relationship between the upper incisors at the pertinent moment, namely the time of eruption.

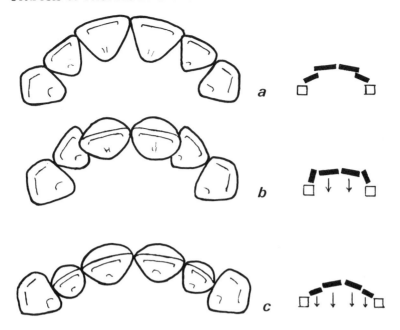

Fig. 11.11. *a*, Upper centrals, mutually supported and normally inclined to base. *b*, Central incisors retroclined, but laterals supported by cupids. *c*, The retroclination of all four upper incisors. The smaller diagrams indicate the relative positions of the upper incisors, near the time of their eruption, in each of the three situations. Tooth size, arch width and tooth relationship each contribute to the opportunity for the upper centrals to become retroclined (*b*) or all four incisors (*c*), under the influence of the lower lip.

Amongst those with Class II division 2 occlusions there are some who possess exceptionally wide upper dental arches, often related to a mandibular arch of normal width, which usually results in buccal crossbite. It is no surprise that many of these individuals develop a division 2 incisor relationship, because the great width to the upper arch across the cuspid region provides space and consequent lack of obstruction against retroclination for all four upper incisors. So long as the conditions of the other two dimensions have been met, the occlusion must become Class II division 2.

It is also found that, in Class II division 2 occlusions, the average size of the incisor teeth is small in all three dimensions when compared to Class I. Although this is an average, it is also true of a high proportion of individual cases. Smaller than average teeth in an average sized dental arch means the probable provision of space sufficient for at least one of the incisors to become retroclined, when prompted by the presence of the other necessary conditions.

There remain those cases of Class II division 2 occlusion which have upper incisor teeth of a size which is commensurate with the population average, in association with an upper arch width which is also of average proportion, or even slightly less than average. In these cases, the upper centrals can become retroclined if the laterals happen to develop in mesio-buccally rotated positions. The laterals escape from their usual developmental positions palatal to the central and, at eruption, fail to support the distal edges of the centrals, thus allowing the lower lip to bring about retroclination of the centrals, if the other conditions needed are also present. The lateral incisors do not retrocline, being supported on their distal aspects by the deciduous and later the permanent cuspids.

The apparent crowding with overlapping of the labial surface of the centrals by the permanent laterals, is not usually seen at the time of eruption, but occurs later with the eruption of the cheek teeth.

Diagrammatic illustration of the three alternative conditions, described above, which relate to the proportional balance of tooth size, arch width and tooth position in the lateral dimension, is provided by *Fig.* 11.11*a*, *b* and *c*.

Overbite

One of the most prevalent characteristics of Class II division 2 occlusions is the presence of deep overbite. The same elements listed as responsible for the promotion of Class II division 2 incisor relationships are also the underlying causes of the deep overbite.

If each of these elements are taken in turn and re-examined for their potential to provide a deep overbite, the following observations can be made:

1. In Class II division 2 occlusions, a combination of mandibular size, posture and lack of posterior dento–alveolar height conspire by variable contributions, to ensure that the inter-maxillary space which the anterior dento–alveolar structures have to cross, when the posterior teeth are in occlusion, is either average, or, much more frequently, less than average, by Class I standards. The space can consequently be crossed anteriorly by alveolar processes of average, or less than average, vertical growth potential;

2. The full vertical potential will be released unless arrested by contact with opposing structures, and

3. The failure, or near failure, of the incisors to contact those of the opposite arch, is ensured by one or other, or a combination of, the following:
   (i) The presence of a Skeletal II dental base relationship;
   (ii) The relatively lingual location of the lower alveolar process through soft tissue moulding; or
   (iii) Moulding which restricts the width of the lower alveolar process, thus limiting the labial inclination of the lower incisors.

The above factors are productive of situations wherein the lower incisors are unlikely to contact the incisal or middle thirds of the crowns of the uppers. If contact is made it will be at or near the cingulum. It is also the case that, when the lower incisors have been compelled to take up an upright position relative to the maxillary structures, a high inter-incisal angle is produced with the palatally inclined upper centrals. Although a statistical correlation can be shown between the depth of overbite and the inter-incisal angle in group analysis, the location of the point of contact of the lower incisor edge on the palatal surface of the uppers and the anatomical form of that surface has more influence on the degree of overbite than the inter-incisal angle. The latter may assist but is not critical.

Figure 11.6e and f contrasts the facial outlines and tooth positions of those ten cases, selected from the now familiar sample of 14-year Class II division 2 occlusions, which possessed the smaller and those ten which showed the greater overbites.

It will be seen that the group with the larger overbites have lower gonial and maxillary–mandibular planes angles and other features, previously given, which are associated with the least labial inclination of the lower incisors (*Fig. 11.6d*). Also present is the strong Skeletal II element associated with the maximum retroclination of the upper incisors (*Fig. 11.6b*). The combination has caused the incisors to almost miss one another on eruption, which is a significant issue in determining the size of the overbite, and, as an incidental by-product of the same factors, a high inter-incisal angle has been formed.

Swallowing

Difficulty in performing the act of swallowing is found almost exclusively in patients with Class II division 1 occlusions. Some such patients, notably those with marked Skeletal II dental base relationships and increased lower face height, with associated large overjets and decreased overbites, together with an inability to comfortably approximate the lips, find it difficult to swallow in the typical manner. They are unable, with these anatomical handicaps, to seal off the front of the mouth, so that the oral fluids can be expelled, without embarrassment, in the appropriate direction. One way by which they overcome their problem is to reflexly move the tongue forward over the lower incisors and against the lower lip, so making an anterior oral seal when swallowing.

It is noticeable that, of those patients who become persistent thumb-suckers, many seem to have these anatomical characteristics. It is tempting to suggest that thumb-sucking in the very young is a perfectly normal conditioned reflex, having its origin in the suckling act, but that, for some, there is a call to extend the process to assist swallowing in adverse anatomical circumstances. Placing the thumb between upper and lower incisors could become a means of assisting an anterior oral seal, as an alternative to the use of the tongue in a similar manner and for the same purpose. It is at least a thought that, for some, thumb-sucking may become a long term habit, less for psychological reasons than from physiological necessity.

Class II division 2 occlusions, on the other hand, are associated with plentiful lip tissue with which to create the necessary oral seal with ease from the earliest age. They do not possess any of the anatomical irregularities listed above and consequently can be expected to abandon thumb-sucking early having no reason to use the tongue or thumb to assist in forming an anterior oral seal.

Conclusion

The development of Class II division 2 occlusions has been given in some detail, partly because of the availability of original research material, but mostly to provide example of the ways by which hard and soft tissue variations can combine to promote an eventual occlusal pattern. Class III and Class II division 1 occlusions also have their subtleties, but their *raison d'etre* is perhaps more readily understood because of the greater contribution made, in their case by the antero–posterior skeletal discrepancy factor.

The formative elements underlying the establishment of Class II division 2 occlusions are less consistent and clear cut. The antero–posterior skeletal discrepancy is mild, and dental bases can be long or short, wide or relatively narrow. The lower arches can be found crowded or otherwise, with lower incisors considerably labially inclined, or alternatively, relatively upright. Lower facial heights can be of normal dimensions, or much reduced. Gonial angles can be high or low, likewise the maxillary–mandibular planes angles. The height of the dento–alveolar structures posteriorly can be average, or reduced with overclosure, when the posterior teeth are in occlusion. Two types of lip pattern can be broadly described which differ notably in appearance. The growth patterns of the mandible can be of either the opening or closing variety.

Within this sea of variation, consistency is only found in the total product. The variables combine, in differing proportions, to produce in each instance:

1. A high lip to upper central incisor relationship;

2. An antero–posterior space between the tips of the lower incisors and those of the erupting uppers; and

3. A lack of mutual buttressing amongst the upper anteriors against the retractive effect of the lower lip upon them.

The formation of Class II division 2 can be regarded as intermediate between that of Class I and Class II division 1.

Some Class I occlusions develop upon a mild Skeletal II base. The small potential overjet is eliminated by a natural compensatory labial inclination of the lower incisors and very minor amounts of upper incisor retraction under the influence of the lower lip. The retraction of the upper incisors, as they erupt, can only be detected by serial lateral skull radiographic study, which covers the area of their eruption. The minority of Class I cases which show $3°-5°$ retroclination of the upper centrals on eruption, can be contrasted with the majority which show the opposite tendency. What is seen in the minority is the beginning of Class II division 2 occlusal formation, in which, if the lower incisor tips were to be less labially inclined, or placed further to the lingual relative to the uppers through one cause or another, the amount of upper central incisor retroclination which would subsequently take place would be greater and would become clinically obvious.

Alternatively, if the upper dental base were to be shortened antero–posteriorly, with no alteration to the labially inclined lower incisors, nor to the slight upper central incisor retroclination, the near Class I case can become classified as Class II division 2 because of the forward position of the upper cheek teeth and the marked prominence of the upper laterals. Such cases usually have a lower facial height of average dimension and no great overlap between lower lip and upper centrals. Occlusions of this kind can be treated without difficulty to high standards of result, because of the absence of any serious skeletal or soft tissue aberrations.

Prognoses for high standards of treatment result diminish as skeletal and soft tissue anomalies increase, particularly in respect of the vertical dimension. The lowered gonial angles, small alveolar heights, mandibular overclosure and a mandibular growth pattern of the closing type, all of which can contribute to small lower face heights, make total elimination of overbite to the edge-to-edge incisor position increasingly difficult and indeed, in the real extreme, probably physically impossible.

Variation antero—posteriorly in the dental base relationship can only be mild for a division 2 incisor relationship to be established, but in terms of the average, the greater the Skeletal II discrepancy, the greater the upper incisor retro-clination and, consequently the greater the mechanical problem of repositioning the upper incisor apices during treatment.

If a dental base relationship is markedly Class II, or the upper incisors happen mutually to support each other against retroclination, the result must be a Class II division 1 occlusion, not division 2.

In the case of some Class II division 1 occlusions, the two conditions of mild Skeletal II relationship and high lip line, necessary to promote division 2, are present, but not the third factor: namely the absence of mutual support amongst the upper anteriors. If the lack of support is introduced by creating space in the upper anterior region by, for example, first bicuspid extraction and subsequent cuspid retraction, all conditions will have been met for the transmutation of one form of malocclusion into the other, if simple retraction of the upper incisors by tilting only is carried out.

Chapter 12

Treatment of Class II division 2

The classification of occlusion, introduced by Dr Edward Angle, was originally based on the relationship between the first permanent molars; but then, with the addition of the incisor relationship, it came to be generally descriptive of the pattern of occlusion as a whole. It is possible, however, for two separate occlusions to fulfil the conditions necessary to be classified fairly as, for example, Class II division 1, yet be quite dissimilar to one another in respect of skeletal form and soft tissue pattern.

The preceding chapter on the development of Class II division 2 and group analysis of developed untreated examples of that form of occlusion was aimed at indicating the extent of variation which is to be found in both the hard and soft tissues surrounding the same pattern of occlusion.

One influence of these variations is upon relative prognosis for treatment. So long as variations in the structures surrounding the dentition are mild, the chances of successful treatment remain good, but once more severe skeletal discrepancies appear, the chances for fully successful outcome deteriorate, no matter what appliance system is to be used. In the worst instances the condition may be beyond the scope of appliances alone to correct, e.g. a Class III occlusion related to an extreme Skeletal III dental base relationship. Surgery has to be considered in such cases.

Another influence of the extensive variation within the surrounding and supporting structures, is upon treatment planning.

Those orthodontists who are either unfamiliar with Stone Age man's attritional dentition theory, or insufficiently convinced of its application to the treatment of present day occlusions, might question whether, in the face of so much variation surrounding Class II division 2, any universal standard treatment procedure, such as is offered by the Begg theory and technique, could always be applied and still give total satisfaction in all possible respects and in every instance.

It is perhaps not so much a question of whether such a standardized form of treatment could be applied on all occasions, but more as to whether it should be. One is bound to be aware of some examples of Class II division 2 occlusions which have been treated by edgewise appliance to give slight distal movement of the upper buccal segments, either with or without the extraction of the upper second molars, using headgear and avoiding interference with a well aligned lower arch. Where such action has been taken in association with long dental bases, the results have been stable and given no cause for complaint. To extract the first permanent molars instead of the second in these cases in order to promote the use of reciprocal intra-oral anchorage, may not always be satisfactory, in that the second molars can be of diminished size resembling third molars, or be of poor quality. Such apparently trivial issues must be given thought before accepting any universal system for treatment.

There also exist a few examples of patients, now well advanced in years, whose facial profile is considered by some to have suffered from the application of the Begg technique by becoming unduly flattened. These treatments have not always been carried out by novices, nor by those wont to tamper with the appliance mechanics by unwarranted modifications of their own. Could it not be that it was the treatment plan which was wrong in these instances? Certainly there would appear to be a grey area lying somewhere between the obvious desirability of extraction in the face of dental overcrowding and the equally desirable avoidance of so doing where both dental arches possess spacing. At exactly what point does it become necessary in theory to compensate for the absence of attrition by the planned removal of teeth? After all, the removal of tooth tissue equivalent to the calculated loss by attrition from certain isolated points within the dental arches is not the same as a gradual loss in small quantities from each unit. Mesial migration of teeth, anterior to the extraction sites, still proceeds and may assist, in conjunction with the anterior overbite, in producing late lower incisor crowding.

Dr Begg's work on the skulls of ancient Australian aboriginals and his theory of the attritional dentition, developed from it, should be studied in full before accepting or rejecting the opinions of those who harbour criticism. His theory has much strength as an explanation of the modern prevalence of dental overcrowding, late lower incisor imbrication and susceptibility to disease of present day dentitions. The question is whether the theory can be extended to justify extraction in orthodontic treatment on almost all occasions.

What seems to be required is not a universal treatment approach which, no matter whether based on extraction or non-extraction, intra-oral or extra-oral anchorage, may fail, by those very restrictions, to give full satisfaction in every instance, but a comprehensive appliance which can be varied to supply the needs of any reasonable tooth movement programme. For this reason one would wish for the recognition of a limited use of headgear with the Begg appliance to cover unusual eventualities created by human variation as a means of avoiding interference with the lower arch where circumstances indicate it.

There are some situations within the treatment of Class II division 2 occlusions, which might reasonably be thought to warrant the use of headgear, although the majority can, and possibly should, be treated by the standard application of the Begg technique.

Whatever the chosen supply of anchorage, the Begg appliance as a mechanism is as efficient as any for carrying out the tooth movements demanded, including the correction of the upper incisor root positions in the Class II division 2 case. Overall treatment times are modest by any standards and chairside time reduced by comparison with other available techniques.

Class II Division 2 Treatment Problems

Correction by appliance of the antero—posterior arch relationship in Class II division 2 should not provide difficulty, since variation in that plane, associated with that form of occlusion, is not great. As was seen in the last chapter, it is the range of variation in the vertical dimension which is, by comparison, much greater and of more practical significance. The variation in the lower face height can range from around the accepted normal to one much reduced, which complicates the incisor relationship and, if really severe, may make full overbite reduction difficult.

The main appliance problems of Class II division 2 treatments lie in the anterior of the mouth and concern the positions of the teeth within, and the relationship between, the labial segments. These could be enumerated as:

1. Difficulties associated with attainment of an edge-to-edge incisor relationship where the lower facial height is severely reduced and where mandibular growth is inadequate, or of the adverse pattern;
2. Difficulties associated with the repositioning of the upper incisor roots, either resulting from item 1 above and/or from premature contact with the palatal wall; and
3. Difficulty arising from a very high inter-incisal angle which has promoted a shearing or scissor-like bite between upper and lower incisors. This can, in conjunction with deep overbite, prevent placement of brackets on the lower incisors, or cause them to be liable to damage in the initial phase of treatment.

The above problems do not arise in every Class II division 2 case, but when present they can cause some difficulty with any appliance. In the case of the standard Begg technique, one additional difficulty should be mentioned which relates to the intrusion of upper incisors. The difficulty arises through the use of Class II inter-maxillary elastics, which, through their vertical components of force, pull downwards on the upper archwire, largely cancelling the intrusive effect of the upper posterior anchor bends on the upper anterior teeth. Increasing the amount of upper anchor bend does not solve the problem, but has the effect of producing excessive distal tilt of the anchor molars, rather than increased intrusion anteriorly. This problem is purely mechanical and is additional to any obstruction to upper incisor intrusion caused, usually in patients with small lower face height, by the proximity of the apices to the floor of the nose.

Obviously, where tooth movement difficulty exists, there may arise the reciprocal problem of the supply of adequate anchorage.

Means of circumventing each of the foregoing

treatment problems will be dealt with in turn, during the description of appliance procedures for the correction of Class II division 2 occlusions.

Practical Approach to the Treatment of Class II Division 2

Many Class II division 2 occlusions present for treatment with an element of dental overcrowding, but no adverse skeletal or other discrepancies so great as to cause them to be exceptions to the application of the standard Begg technique.

Extractions can be carried out to provide space for accommodation of the teeth in their corrected positions and for the associated foreseeable controlled movement of the anchor units. The factors governing the choice of units for extraction do not differ from those already described when discussing the treatment of Class II division 1 (*see* Chapter 9).

Following on extraction, Stages 1, 2 and 3 of the standard Begg technique can be used, with no additions or subtractions, in exactly the same basic manner as described for the treatment of Class II division 1. Of course, in the case of division 2, the objectives in the upper incisor region are a little different, in that there will be less crown retraction and more palatal movement of the apices demanded by the nature of the untreated condition. Apical movements make a relatively high demand on anchorage, a fact which must be taken into account when planning the balance of anchorage through choice of extraction in the first instance.

The many published case reports showing treatment of the Class II division 2 form of occlusion using the Begg appliance and technique, bear testimony to its efficiency in the circumstances. It is seldom, however, that such reports include cases where the original prognosis was poor, owing to the presence of one or other of the adverse factors mentioned above. When such cases are shown, they can be expected to be those with successful outcome, their authors knowing that more has been achieved than could reasonably have been expected having regard to the original condition. In all probability, the fortuitous advent of favourable growth alone will have converted a modest standard of result into the spectacular: in reality an orthodontist can do no more than use his appliance correctly and to the full. In adverse circumstances this may not always be enough to obtain the perfect result, but this fact must not become a general excuse for not aiming at perfection: defeat should not be accepted unless it becomes genuinely unavoidable.

Overbite Reduction

The desired edge-to-edge incisor relationship can be obtained in a high percentage of Class II division 2 occlusions through the use of the standard Begg technique. In those cases which present variable amounts of difficulty because of unfavourable mandibular growth patterns and related small lower face heights, any of the mechanical measures for obtaining the maximum intrusive effects from the archwires, outlined in Chapter 8, can be used. These include the use of posterior vertical elastics, possible banding of second molars, and the application of labial root torque on the lower incisors. The purpose and method of these additions do not differ in the case of Class II division 2 from the description already given. In the most severely increased overbites, however, maximum possible intrusion of the lower anteriors only may not be enough to gain an edge-to-edge incisor relationship. Some intrusion of the upper incisors, possibly also to the maximum possible extent, will be needed. Such intrusion in Class II division 2 would appear desirable, in that the upper incisors will be brought up from within the lower lip, so reducing the amount of lip to upper incisor overlap.

The amount of upper incisor intrusion resulting from the standard application of the Begg technique is not great, because the inter-maxillary elastics offset the intrusive effect of the upper archwire on the anteriors. This means that the Begg technique, in its purest form, must be altered, if only for a short period, during the course of treatment.

In order to improve the posterior vertical anchorage, the first permanent molars can be supported against distal tilt by inclusion of the second molars in the band-up. Alternatively, similar support and elevation of the first molars can be given by the use of posterior vertical elastics between hooks on the disto–buccal of the upper and lower molars each side. The archwires should be 0·018 in or 0·020 in and, for the time being, the use of Class II elastics should be discontinued. These actions amount to an additional stage devoted to bite opening only and would be instituted as a part of a Stage 1 in which an unsatisfactory amount of overbite reduction had been achieved.

As a final alternative, to be applied at the same point in treatment before the extraction spaces become finally closed, high pull headgear can be used to assist upper incisor intrusion, in conjunction with the conventional posterior anchor bend. The headgear is applied to rings, incorporated into the archwire mesial to the upper laterals, which are additional to the conventional hooks, or rings, mesial to the cuspids. Class II elastics may have to be temporarily discontinued until the bite has opened. Headgear force should not exceed 250 g (see Chapter 8).

Note should be taken, prior to and during intrusion of upper incisors, of the location of the apices relative to the nasal floor. In low anterior facial heights, the alveolar vertical dimension will be small, in consequence of which there may be little bone above the upper central incisor apices available for intrusion before the obstruction of the nasal floor is reached. Ideally, the ultimate object will be to torque the central incisor apices palatally, not only for improvement of the interincisal angle, but also to angle them away from the floor of the nose into the area of convergence between the palatal wall and the nasal floor which gives the optimum possibility of intrusion. Normally this would be a part of Stage 3 objectives.

In the case of upper incisor intrusion by high pull headgear, however, there is the theoretical threat of causing further apical displacement of the upper centrals labially. For this reason, it is often advisable to fit a palatal root torque auxiliary, gently active, during the separate bite opening phase, in order to provide axial control and to begin to move the upper central incisor apices towards their intended destination. The process may temporarily create a mild Class II division 1 appearance, but once the bite is sufficiently reduced the standard Begg procedures can be reinstituted to conclude Stage 1 and the remainder of the treatment, so long as adequate space remains in the extraction sites. The upper archwire should not be turned round the distal of the buccal tubes when the headgear is being worn, because to do so would be both unnecessary and also liable to bring the upper buccal teeth forward, if the overjet should temporarily increase.

It must also be noted that it may not always be possible to move the upper incisor apices as far palatally as one might wish, if the palatal wall is steep and contact is made prematurely between it and some part of the incisor roots. Once such contact is made, continuation of the torque action may cause root resorbtion and begin to reintroduce an overjet as the roots are levered against the palatal wall. Interference from the palatal wall will limit the extent of palatal root torque no matter by what means, or at what stage, it is carried out.

The last item of the unusual concerns the presence of a shearing bite, either between the lower incisors and the two upper centrals, or all four upper incisors. This must be eliminated before brackets can be placed on the lower incisors without risk of damage to the upper incisal edges or the lower brackets themselves.

Where this problem is provided by the upper centrals only, it is usual to find that the upper laterals are relatively labially inclined and prominent. In this situation the placement of an upper alignment archwire will immediately bring the crowns of the centrals labially into line with those of the laterals, thereby creating the space needed for the fitting of the lower incisor brackets, after which the standard Stage 1 mechanics can proceed.

The problem of the shearing bite will be more difficult to overcome if all four upper incisors are not only retroclined, but also well aligned. Since, in this instance, there are no prominent laterals, or cuspids, alignment by plain archwire may not produce adequate clearance for the safe placement of lower incisor brackets.

One possible answer, is to fit an 0·018 in or 0·020 in conventional Stage 1 upper archwire, to which is added an anterior active palatal root torque auxiliary. The reciprocal effect of the root torque will be to move the upper incisor crowns labially, so that a mild overjet is formed and, at the same time, space gained for the banding of the lower arch including the incisors. A lower Stage 1 archwire is then fitted. Once both archwires are in position, posterior vertical elastics and/or high pull headgear can be used until the bite has fully opened. Standard Stage 1 mechanics cannot be applied until this has happened, because the removal of the upper torque auxiliary would permit the upper incisors to tilt back once more into a shearing relationship with the lowers. To leave the upper torque auxiliary in place and retract bodily would be expensive in lower arch anchorage.

It follows from the above that, where there is an inter-incisal scissor-like bite which prevents the immediate commencement of lower arch treatment, the separate bite opening stage must be instituted at the very commencement of Stage 1.

So much has been written in this chapter concerning the unusual within the treatment of Class II division 2, that the reader may have gained a warped impression of the balance of usage of the Begg appliance for the correction of this class of occlusion. It should be remembered that the basic Begg technique will satisfy all requirements for the majority of cases. The apparent lack of balance in the description, is due to the fact that it has been thought unnecessary to repeat the detail of basic procedures which have already been covered in dealing with the treatment of Class II division 1.

Anchorage

The amount of lower arch anchorage available in any given case can also be judged from the principles given under the treatment of division 1. It so happens that the lower incisors in some Class II division 2 cases are housed in an alveolar process which is narrow antero–posteriorly. This will improve lower arch anchorage for these individuals by providing a natural control against labial tilting of the lower incisors. Where no such natural control exists, it can be partially provided artificially by the application of a lower incisor labial root torque auxiliary.

When monitoring the position of the lower labial segment radiographically during the course of treatment, it may be found, usually in low gonial angle cases, that the angle between the SN line and lower central incisor edges (SNIL) has increased to an extent that, if the lower incisor tip movement were alone responsible, the future stability of the lower incisors would be in doubt. In many such instances, however, closer inspection may reveal that all points on the lower symphyseal cross-section have moved forward in relation to the Nasion to the same degree as the incisor edges, indicating that the tooth movement is related to general mandibular growth. This means that the lower incisor crowns have not altered their position relative to the lower lip which, from the point of view of their ultimate stability, is very different from having moved the crowns into the lip tissue.

Use of the APo or Holdaway lines will reveal which of the two events has taken place. SNI measurement should never be used as the sole manner of assessing potential changes in the lower incisor position.

If, through radiographic assessment, it is discovered towards the conclusion of treatment of a Class II division 2 occlusion that lower arch anchorage has been expended, but it remains desirable and possible to continue palatal apical movement of the upper incisors, the upper arch can be supported against labial shift by employing headgear, whilst Class II mechanics are discontinued. It is probably better to apply the headgear arms to the anterior of the upper archwire, rather than applying the force through a Kloehn type facebow fitted into supplementary buccal tubes on the molars.

The use of headgear to supply anchorage for the conclusion of the treatment where lower arch anchorage has been spent would be preferable to indulging in further extraction for the same purpose, particularly if the loss of the lower anchorage is associated with an error of judgement or mechanics on the part of the operator. The infallible orthodontist is, after all, a fictitious character. Mistakes, however, in the comparatively slow moving business of tooth movement, should never be allowed to reach the point at which they become irretrievable. The use of headgear, in the above context, offers an effective means of retrieving a situation and requires an upper archwire with rings for the attachment of the headgear arms in the lateral incisor region together with an increased curve of Spee. It must be admitted that patient cooperation with headgear at a late stage in treatment is, on the whole, less easily obtained than at the outset and consequently needs more than ever the support of a sound logical argument in its favour to gain the patient's interest.

Non-Extraction Treatment

General spacing of the dental arches is sometimes a feature of Class II division 1 occlusions, but, by the nature of things, it most unlikely to be found in division 2. It is therefore the case that, where anchorage is required in any quantity, which will be almost certainly so in the correction of division 2 occlusions, anchorage supply for a non-extraction approach must come from extra-oral sources. In spite of arguments in favour of extraction, it is still worth considering a non-extraction approach for the few Class II division 2 cases which do not possess crowding of the lower arch, have mild increase of overbite, long dental bases and only slight displacement of the upper central incisor apices labially, but some labial displacement of the crowns of the laterals, supported by a quarter to half a unit Class II relationship of the buccal teeth. In such a situation, distal movement of the upper molars using a Kloehn bow to double molar tubes can be followed by the use of Begg appliance components fitted to all teeth mesial to the first molars, to retract, align, then correct the root positions where necessary. This, although representing a complete digression from the Begg theory and technique, could, so long as the case selected is appropriate, save time and teeth.

Chapter 13

Treatment of Class III

An occlusion which can be classified as Angle's Class I is accepted by the dental profession as that which is nearest to the ideal from the points of view of function and prevention and is equally acceptable, not only to the profession but to the lay public, as often representative of the best in aesthetic appearance. An ideal occlusion, however, can only be expected to develop when the dental, skeletal and soft tissue facial elements are well balanced, showing only modest degrees of variation.

Class II division 2 represents the first clear step away from the Class I ideal. Variation in the structures surrounding and supporting that form of occlusion are manifold, but not always severe, allowing many to be treated to a high standard of result. When severity does enter, it usually concerns the vertical dimension and, occasionally, the lateral. Antero—posterior discrepancies are mild and the upper anteriors are able to erupt within the confines of the lips, through which natural compensation is provided for the potential overjet, causing palatal tilt of upper incisors and varying degrees of labial tilt of the lowers.

If Class I and Class II division 2 occlusions can be regarded as a middle range, Class II division 1 and Class III lie left and right of this centre having, in addition to vertical and lateral proportional skeletal discrepancies, a far stronger tendency to extremes in the antero—posterior dimension.

In the case of Class III, the situation of reverse overjet is created either by suitable aberration of the upper and lower incisor positions, or through a malrelationship of maxilla to mandible, or by a combination of the two. The maxilla can be proportionately small in relation to a mandible of normal size, or the mandible relatively large in proportion to a maxilla of normal size. A lack of coordination between the size of the maxilla and mandible can also produce buccal crossbite, either unilaterally or bilaterally.

The size of gonial angle within Class III is variable and contains examples of both the high and the low, which are in turn loosely associated with increase and decrease of the lower facial height and incisor overbite. Lower dental base lengths tend to be either average or above average, but the lengths of upper dental bases show a full range of variation from short to long, creating a condition for either the absence of crowding of the upper teeth, or the reverse.

Once again, occlusions warranting the same occlusal classification, can be associated with supporting and surrounding structures which show considerable differences from one case to another. In Class III, as in Class II division 2, these differences might reasonably be expected to have some influence on both treatment planning and prognosis.

Using his mechanical appliances the orthodontist can modify the position of the individual teeth within the limits set by the supporting bone and surrounding soft tissues. The position and shape of the alveolar processes are not greatly affected by his exertions and his direct influence on the elements of the main skeleton appears to be even less.

Where Class III reverse overjet is created by appropriate malplacement of the upper and lower incisors, and/or the contribution made by the skeletal factor is mild, correction by appliance will provide little difficulty.

Some such cases may appear more severe than they actually are, in that patients who are not quite able to occlude their teeth with the incisors in the correct relationship have to adopt a forward posture of the mandible on closure. In the closed position, the forward displacement of the mandible worsens appearance in profile.

The displacement element can be clinically assessed by inducing the patient to place his anterior teeth in as near to normal relationship as possible. Many Class III patients will manage an edge-to-edge, or near edge-to-edge, incisor relationship, but some will be found unable, by variable amounts, to approach such a position. Extreme examples of the latter represent the more severe conditions which may be untreatable by orthodontic measures alone.

If the patient can approximate his anterior teeth in near edge-to-edge relationship, the amount of adjustment needed to produce a correct incisor relationship can be judged clinically. Lateral skull radiographs, taken prior to treatment and also in the edge-to-edge position, can be of service in determining more precisely not only the degree of correction needed, but also the inter-incisal angle which will result.

It is important to see that bone is available in sufficient quantity in the areas to which the teeth are to be moved and that, after movement, their new relationship will be both aesthetically satisfactory and atraumatic.

The correction of reverse overjet is usually expedited by moving the opposed teeth of both arches rather than of just one. By a combination of lingual tilting of the lower incisors and, at the same time, a proclination of the uppers, mild degree reverse overjets can quickly be corrected, with a shortening of the traumatic interlude which can occur at the point where the teeth are 'neither here nor there'.

The same practical approach can be used when correcting buccal crossbite, which is not infrequently associated with Class III occlusions, unilaterally or bilaterally. Correction will be expedited by combining lateral expansion of the upper arch with a measure of contraction of the lower. In cases where it is deemed undesirable to actually cause contraction of the lower arch, the presence of a passive lower archwire will prevent the lower buccal teeth from responding to upper arch expansion by themselves moving bucally. Cuspal conflict and interlocking can produce this latter movement unless prevented.

So long as reverse overjet or buccal crossbite are associated with tooth malplacement or tilt, appliance correction is possible; but in many instances these occlusal deformations are related, in variable degree, to either antero–posterior or lateral discrepancies within the supporting skeleton. Orthodontic tooth movements cannot compensate for more than modest discrepancies in relative shape, size, and relationship between the mandibular and maxillary dental bases, and still have the expectation of a sound functional result. It is up to the orthodontist to judge whether, in the case of the individual, bodily movement or tilting of the teeth in appropriate directions and within their bony confines can promote compensation for skeletal imbalance and at the same time produce a more functional relationship between the teeth than that which already exists.

Some crossbites may have to be accepted and some more extreme reverse overjets may need to be considered in the light of possible surgical intervention. In these latter instances, orthodontic treatment and bite rehabilitation may still be needed in conjunction with the surgery.

Overbite

The amount of anterior overbite encountered in the untreated Class III case varies considerably, ranging from those individuals showing a marked increase, to those who exhibit a decrease which amount to anterior open bite.

The deeper anterior overbites are usually, but not always, associated with smaller than average heights of the lower third of the face and low Frankfurt–mandibular (FM) plane angles, whilst the decreased or open bite cases are associated, in the main, with the opposite conditions. In cases where the vertical height to the lower face is unusually great, the potential to further vertical alveolar development may be already exhausted, in which case mechanical closure may prove difficult or actually impossible, unlike open bites associated with a stultification of alveolar development by, for example, the intrusion of thumb or finger.

The establishment of a positive overbite by the conclusion of treatment, is undoubtedly desirable, wherever it can be achieved, for the stability of the corrected incisor relationship. In different Class III occlusions there may be a call for some overbite reduction, or the maintainance of the existing amount, or an actual increase in the existing amount. It is an unfortunate fact that, where a positive overbite is so desirable and where, in the context of high facial heights and high FM plane angles, it may be difficult to obtain: growth directions, or amounts, will so frequently prove disadvantageous. It can happen that positive overbites, established at the conclusion of treatment, may later disappear as a result of the vertical component of facial growth.

The orthodontic treatment of Class III occlusions is therefore not without its limitations and will consist of the correction of reverse overjet together with the establishment of a positive incisor overbite wherever possible. It will also include the correction of any buccal crossbite and the elimination of tooth displacements through crowding, wherever these feature, whilst at the same time making the best of the occlusal relationships of the buccal teeth antero–posteriorly.

Dental Overcrowding and Extraction in Class III Occlusions

Because the mandibles of patients with Class III occlusions tend to be of average, or above average size, the manifestations of dental crowding in the lower arch are less common than in the upper, where there is a greater tendency to a relatively restricted dental base. Extraction of units to relieve crowding are consequently more probable in the upper arch, but the fact that the lower labial segment will usually need to be retracted in order to establish the proper inter-incisal relationship may demand creation of space for this purpose, unless already there by nature. It should also be noted that levelling of the lower dental arch and lower incisor depression also requires space. If the teeth of the lower arch are in firm proximal contact, well aligned but in need of some incisor depression, the act of levelling will lengthen the arch with slight labial movement of the incisors. This must be kept in mind when planning any treatment, as must be the fact that, in Class III, the upper anteriors will usually be moved labially which will assist in reducing the amount of crowding of the upper arch present at the outset.

If extractions are to be carried out, the units removed will be those which provide the best balance of anchorage to back the subsequent tooth movements for each individual. Where the teeth of the upper arch, particularly the labial segment, exhibit gross malplacement labio–palatally, or rotation, the teeth to be extracted will probably be the first bicuspids. The same teeth will equally probably be removed from lower arches, where there is evidence of some overcrowding and/or there is a need for maximum possible retraction of the lower labial segment.

The milder the original condition, the less posterior anchorage will be required, allowing the extraction sites to be placed further posteriorly in the second bicuspid or first molar regions.

The preservation of the upper first bicuspids,

when possible, assists the stability of the upper labial segment in its corrected position by providing buccal segment tooth support as an addition to the factor of positive overbite. Where the upper first bicuspids have to be sacrificed, subsequent space closure and root reorientation should be fully carried through, so as to ensure the same buccal segment support to the upper anteriors.

When it is remembered that there may be, in certain instances, a congenital absence of some teeth in Class III cases and that the wish to preserve the upper first bicuspids can lead to the choice for extraction of upper second bicuspids and lower first, it becomes apparent that the appliance mechanics should be adjustable to handle the result of practically any possible combination of extractions.

The Begg appliance has the required versatility. It is also, with its ability to increase the posterior or anterior anchorage resistance at will, an excellent mechanism for the closure of large amounts of unwanted space. This ability is frequently needed in the treatment of the lower arch in Class III occlusions, particularly where it has been deemed advisable to extract the first bicuspids in order to be able to retract the lower labial segment to the maximum extent. It will be found that the amount by which the lower labial segment can be retracted, even after the removal of first lower bicuspids, is restricted by the lingual cortical plate. Initially the lower incisor crowns respond to Class III elastics, or a lower intra-maxillary force, by moving lingually with little labial transference of their root ends, but as they tilt they become obstructed by the lingual cortical plate which forms a fulcrum near the necks of the teeth. Thereafter, continuation of the applied force produces little additional lingual movement of the crowns, but proportionately more labial apical shift. This undesirable root movement may, in some cases, have to be limited by the application of a lower lingual root torque auxiliary (see Fig. 13.5). The same lingual root torque will assist the anchorage resistance of the lower labial segment against the pull of lower intra-maxillary and Class III inter-maxillary elastics, thus making possible the closure of considerable first bicuspid extraction space mainly by the mesial movement of the posteriors. The closure of comparatively large amounts of residual extraction space in the lower arch of Class III cases, following first bicuspid removal, is more readily and speedily carried out by the Begg appliance than by others employing bodily movement principles.

Finally, there are undoubtedly examples of Class III occlusions which can and should be treated without resort to extraction. For the most part these will be the milder cases, showing minimal crowding effects in the upper arch and none in the lower. The simple labial movement of the upper incisors will promote the space required for the alignment of those teeth and, at the same time, create a positive overjet which, with minimal retraction of the lower anteriors, produces a positive atraumatic overbite and inter-incisal relationship.

The varied circumstances surrounding the Class III form of occlusion should be thoroughly assessed before deciding on a treatment programme. It is surely unwise, in the face of all the possible variations, to approach treatment blindfolded by adherence to any routine system. The reflex removal of the first bicuspids, followed by a three stage mechanical treatment with the Begg appliance, whilst being entirely successful in some contexts, can, nevertheless, in other less propitious circumstances lead to a protracted treatment largely devoted to space closure. At worst, the final outcome can look very like the original occlusion, except that four teeth have been removed. It should also be noted that, in the treatment of Class III as elsewhere, some consideration should be given to the possible effects of extractions on the facial profile.

The suggestion of a non-extraction approach for some individuals would appear to flaunt the theory of attritional dentition. Here, as has been explained elsewhere in this text, (*see* pp. 96–98) the suggestion is made on the ground of what the author believes to be practical reality.

Mechanics for the Treatment of Class III Occlusions

The movement of teeth suited to the correction of Class III occlusions using the Begg appliance can be divided into three stages, as with treatment for other types of occlusion.

The aims of Stage 1 would be:
1. General alignment of the teeth of both arches;
2. Correction of reverse overjet (and buccal crossbite, if present); and
3. Reduction of increased overbite, if required.

Stage 2 involves the completion of space closure and Stage 3 the reorientation of roots, in order to upright any teeth which have become tilted.

As with the treatment of other forms of occlusion, it is a sound general principle that the aims of one stage be fully completed before the next is begun. The aims themselves look, on paper, to be very similar to those applicable to Class II division 1, but, due to the composition of Class III, the practical appliance mechanics are almost the obverse.

Class III inter-maxillary elastics will be used, rather than Class II. The lower incisors will be retracted, not the uppers, the latter being moved labially. If root torque is required for the upper incisors in Stage 3, it will probably be labial rather than palatal. In this connection it will have been noticed that the Stage 1 aims in the case of a Class III occlusion did not include the attainment of an edge-to-edge incisor relationship. The aim instead will be an overbite of normal proportions. In case there should be those who do not appreciate the reason why an edge-to-edge incisor relationship is not a target in Class III treatments, it might be pointed out that in the treatment of Class II, more often than not, a persistent deep overbite is being fought, whereas in Class III the problem will usually be that of obtaining a positive overbite, even where before treatment an overbite was present.

The attainment of an edge-to-edge incisor relationship in the treatment of Class II represents a deliberate over-treatment of the overbite and, at the same time, enables the adjustment of the inter-incisal angle by palatal root movement of the upper anteriors without accompanying labial movement of their crowns. The latter undesirable effect is innevitable if the incisor overbite has been insufficiently reduced.

In the Class III cases, however, the labial movement of the upper anteriors will result in some overbite reduction for which there will usually be an inadequate compensatory increase through the limited lingual movement of the lowers, leaving, on balance, an overall overbite reduction. This reduction in high gonial angle cases, can be more than one would wish, actually creating an anterior open bite. In low gonial angle cases with small lower face heights, the same degree of overbite reduction results in the retention of a normal overlap of the incisors, upper to lower, after correction of the reverse overjet. In this type of individual there may be, at the same point in treatment, a measure of buccal open bite for which correction will come more from posterior vertical development than incisor depression.

Where positive overbite can be achieved, the amount is not of concern in relation to upper incisor root correction, as it is in Class II, because if root torque is required at all, it will most probably be in the labial direction which, by reaction, brings the tips of the upper incisors towards the lowers. In contrast to palatal root movement of the upper incisors, labial root torque can be applied without detriment in the presence of overbite.

As far as Stage 2 space closure is concerned, an opportunity is presented to clarify a general point in respect of the effects of anchorage reversal. Whether the occlusion under treatment is Class III, or some other form, the closure of large amounts of residual space by mesial movement of the posteriors will require the fitting of anterior lingual root torque auxiliaries and/or uprighting springs for distal movement of the cuspid roots, in order to increase the anchorage resistance of the labial segments. Once the auxiliaries have been fitted, the balance of movement will favour the posteriors, so long as they have been kept free to respond; but this does not mean that the anteriors have been completely immobilized. Not only will the projected root movements of the anteriors take place, but also some retraction of the labial segments, albeit bodily, can be expected in response to inter- or intra-maxillary space closing elastics, or similar forces. This fact is not always brought into the equation when calculating the probable total effect of orthodontic treatments on the facial profile.

At the conclusion of Stage 2, when occlusal relationships have been corrected, it will be found in Class III cases that the lower labial segment is, by variable degrees, lingually inclined. It is tempting, in the circumstances, to apply lingual root torque to the lower incisors and to upright the lower cuspids. If this is attempted, it will usually be found that little uprighting of the lower incisors can be accomplished before the tips begin to move labially, through leverage of the roots against the lingual plate, thus threatening to reintroduce the former Class III inter-incisal relationship. At the same time, the lower incisors may take up a less advantageous angle in relation to the labially inclined uppers. Labial root torque would have to be supplied to the latter to avoid the relationship becoming traumatic. In practice, it will be found necessary to accept a measure of lower incisor lingual tilt and, with it, a corresponding distal tilt to the lower cuspids. The full paralleling of the lower cuspid and bicuspid roots should be avoided because, if done, the result can only be an unstable contact relationship between cuspid and lower lateral.

Preliminary or Preparatory Treatment

It may be necessary, for the treatment of those Class III occlusions which are associated with severe antero–posterior skeletal discrepancies, to resort to surgery. Any pre- or post-operative orthodontic movements planned to coordinate with the surgery, will tend to vary from one individual to another, both quantitatively and qualitatively. It is consequently impossible to describe a precise mechanical approach which would be universally applicable. It will be the task of the orthodontist to devise mechanics suited to each individual problem using his knowledge of the basic governing principles of the appliance.

Outside surgery, another form of preliminary treatment quite commonly needed in Class III is for the correction of bilateral crossbite. As with reverse overjet, buccal crossbites can be associated with either tooth malplacement, or skeletal discrepancy, or both. Large amounts of upper arch expansion can be most readily obtained by using a specialized appliance designed for the purpose, prior to extraction or any other action connected with the main treatment. An upper fixed appliance, with incorporated strong expansion screw, is suited to the purpose, and is used on the rapid expansion principle to bring about the required arch enlargement in weeks rather than months (*Fig.* 13.1). When used in this rapid manner, the median suture will be opened and a diastema between the upper centrals may appear. The latter phenomenon is temporary and the gap can be expected to close spontaneously and quickly.

It is not advisable to use rapid palate splitting expansion on older patients, those of sixteen years of age and upwards. The median suture may not separate and pain may be caused.

Unfortunately, as with other, slower forms of arch expansion, the results are not renowned for their stability, particularly immediately following

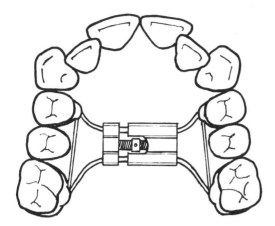

Fig. 13.1. Appliance for rapid expansion of the upper arch and correction of buccal crossbite.

the action. The appliance itself should be left passive in situ as a retainer until the anterior teeth have settled. Once this has been discarded, the appliance for the purpose of the main treatment must be fitted with the minimum of delay. It would be advisable to consider slight expansion to the upper archwire of the new appliance as a safeguard against relapse during the early stages of the main treatment.

Buccal crossbites are often associated with a degree of mandibular displacement, to one side or the other, on closure. This can be detected clinically prior to treatment and will usually rectify as a consequence of upper lateral expansion. There are, however, cases where unilateral crossbite is associated with minor mandibular asymmetry. The dental arches of such individuals may be well formed and symmetrical, but the patient occludes directly into crossbite with no displacement. Since many such cases are Class III, it is a possible thought that the condition may have been promoted by the early establishment of a bite of convenience to avoid obstruction from teeth in the deciduous dentition and that, at this time, compensation occurred through unilateral condylar growth, although not of the progressive variety. This type of crossbite must be differentiated from other kinds, because it does not respond readily to treatment, and so may have to be accepted.

Main Treatment Mechanics

There will doubtless be those orthodontists who will be looking for precise illustration and in-

struction on the archwire forms and adjustments suited to each stage of every known permutation of variation within Class III occlusions. It is not possible, and probably not advisable, to offer anything as comprehensive within a reasonable space. The greatest variation and consequently most numerous mechanical alternatives will be found in the Stage 1 procedures, where the mechanics will be influenced by differing choice of extraction or non-extraction and by the degree of tooth malplacement at the outset of treatment.

In order to show the majority of the mechanical principles and typical archwire forms used for the treatment of Class III, the case chosen is one showing an increased incisor overbite and considerable crowding in the upper labial segment with the upper laterals trapped on the palatal side of the centrals. This upper arch crowding and the need for maximum lower labial segment retraction, has justified the extraction of the four first bicuspids.

Stage 1 Lower Archwires

In the absence of any notable tooth displacements, there will probably be no call for a looped archwire. The lower archwire would therefore be plain and of a pattern already familiar from the treatment of Class II occlusions. Anchor bends would be incorporated just distal to the second bicuspid brackets and, since some overbite reduction is needed, the degree of bend would cause the labial section of the archwire to lie in the buccal sulcus when unpinned. The force required to elevate the anterior section to the level of the bracket slots, should be around 60 g. (*Fig.* 13.2).

If no overbite reduction has been required, the degree of anchor bend would be reduced so as to offer no more than bodily control over the molars as these teeth were moved mesially, i.e. 10° to 15°.

The usual inter-maxillary hook or ring is incorporated, just mesial to the lower cuspid brackets. These hooks will hold the Class III elastics, stretched from the buccal hooks on the upper first molars.

When extractions have been performed in the lower arch of Class III cases, there will almost certainly be superfluous space for all purposes within that arch; consequently lower intra-maxillary elastics can be used in Stage 1 to assist space closure through the mesial movement of the molars.

Class III and intra-maxillary elastics should apply no more than 60 g each.

Stage 1 Upper Archwires

There is more variety of possible tooth position in the Class III upper arch than the lower, which makes for corresponding variations of archwire designs. In the example illustrated, the lateral incisors are locked palatally and there would be

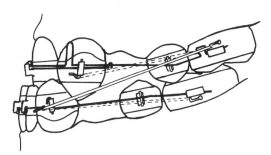

Fig. 13.2. Class III malocclusion with crowded upper labial segment. Upper left and right 1s are moved labially by compressed vertical loop, with the reciprocal force delivered to the molars through stop loops placed against the mesial of the buccal tubes. The supplementary archwire assists stability against canine expansion and the opening of too much space anteriorly. Upper canine retraction, if needed, can be by upper intra-maxillary elastic.

inadequate space between the upper cuspids to allow upper centrals and laterals to be moved labially *en bloc* into a proper relationship to the lower incisors.

In these circumstances, of the alternatives available the approach which produces the quickest results is to move the upper centrals labially over the lower incisors, leaving the upper laterals disconnected from the archwire. The labial movement of the centrals will create space for the accommodation of the laterals, which can then be brought into the line of the arch and also over the lower incisors. In some instances, however, accommodation of the laterals may not be possible without some accompanying distal movement of the upper cuspids. When Class III, rather than Class II, elastics are being worn, the upper cuspids do not show the same tendency to retract spontaneously and, if their distal movement is required, another force for that purpose will have to be introduced.

An upper archwire suited to all the above purposes is shown in *Fig.* 13.2. It contains an

active vertical loop in 0·016 in wire, which creates an antero–posterior expansion force. The anterior section of the archwire, before pinning, will lie just to the labial of the upper central incisor brackets, but, in order that the loop become compressed when pinned anteriorly, there must be a posterior stop loop. In *Fig.* 13.2 the stop is shown against the mesial of the molar tube. An antero–posterior upper arch expansion system is thus set up, but distal movement of the upper molars is unlikely

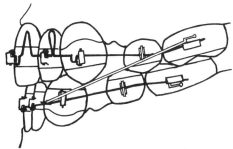

Fig. 13.3. Repositioning of upper lateral incisors by looped archwire. Stops against centrals and cuspids prevent closure of space when lateral incisors are obstructed in labial movement by overbite.

because of the counter pull of the Class III intermaxillary elastics. The labial movement of the centrals is reinforced by the same means. If some retraction of the cuspids is required, an upper intra-maxillary elastic can be applied, exerting 30 to 40 g, between the molars and cuspid pin tags. The reciprocal pull on the molars in a mesial direction would also reinforce the movement of the centrals labially.

If the sprung loop is placed to the mesial of the cuspids it can be used as a hook in the very unlikely event of the need arising for the use of Class II elastics. Another approach, which might suit some occasions, is to place a stop against the mesial of the cuspid brackets instead of the molar. The cuspids will act as anchorage, and will be moved distally at the same time as the centrals respond to the active loop, by moving labially. The space required for the laterals will thus be created. The Class III elastics are able, with this arrangement, to commence mesial movement of the upper posteriors immediately, without obstruction.

When the central incisor positions have been corrected and the space for the laterals opened, a looped archwire can be introduced to complete upper labial segment alignment (*Fig.* 13.3). In a situation where there exists a deep overbite

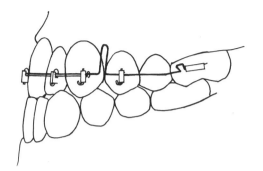

Fig. 13.4. The labial movement of an intact and well aligned upper labial segment. The supplementary archwire prevents anterior spacing and, by being slightly contracted, offsets canine expansion.

between the lower incisors and the upper laterals which are to be brought into line, it is prudent to incorporate lugs into the archwire to contact the distal of the central incisor bracket and the mesial of that of the cuspid. The vertical alignment loops should be kept mildly expanded, in order to prevent possible premature closure of the spaces for the laterals. If this is not done, inadvertant space closure can occur as a result of the obstruction to the labial movement of the laterals from the overbite of the lower incisors. Because of the obstruction, the active loops fail to move the upper laterals fully into line but instead bring upper centrals and cuspids palatally, at the same time reducing the space between them, which subsequently has to be reopened. No such precaution would be needed where overbite is minimal or non-existent.

In the majority of Class III cases, less upper arch crowding will be found than that in the foregoing example. Where displacement of the teeth of the upper incisors is minimal, initial alignment can be obtained with a plain 0·016 in upper archwire, with stops against the molar buccal tubes. When aligned but still in Class III relationship to the lower incisors, or if well aligned before treatment was started, a mechanical system would be needed to move the whole of the upper labial segment labially as a unit. A possible method is shown in *Fig.* 13.4.

When a well aligned upper labial segment is moved to the labial and over the lower incisors, there will be a strong tendency for the segment to become spaced. In the example given in *Fig.* 13.4 a supplementary archwire, looped onto the main, immediately posterior to the cuspid brackets,

keeps the upper anteriors from spacing out and, at the same time, gives additional stability to the anterior of the main archwire against unintentional expansion of the inter-cuspid width.

Space Closure in Treatment of Class III
Stage 2 Archwires

Whenever the treatment of Class III occlusion is based on extraction, there will almost invariably be residual space left in the extraction sites after completion of general tooth alignment and correction of the labial segment relationship. If, through a misjudgement, the extractions have been performed in the wrong area of the dental arches, or have been carried out when a non-extraction approach would have been more appropriate, the most probable result will be the need to close excessive amounts of space, which is not only time consuming, but liable to provide anchorage problems. The problems may be difficult to counter and consequently the standard of the final outcome is threatened.

The Stage 2 archwires are of a conventional pattern similar to those used in the treatment of other forms of malocclusion. 0·018 in or 0·020 in wires are used, carrying the usual inter-maxillary hooks or rings and minimal degree anchor bends combined with slight toe-in. In the Class III case there will seldom be a need to supply forces to maintain overbite reduction, so that the anchor bends should be no greater than that which is required to prevent molar tilt as these teeth are moved mesially. The toe-in bend will prevent the tendency for the molars to rotate mesio—lingually.

The typical Stage 2 mechanical arrangement is shown in *Fig.* 13.5. Class III and lower intra-maxillary space closing elastics are shown in position. In the majority of Class III treatments, completion of the usual elastic complex by the addition of upper intra-maxillary rubbers, should be avoided, so as to eliminate the risk of reintroducing a Class III incisor relationship. The risk would be real, even if the incisor overbite was of normal proportions, but obviously greater if the overbite is only just positive or actually negative.

The use of palatal root torque to the upper incisors as a means of increasing anterior anchorage resistance will seldom be applicable to the Class III case which, by this stage in treatment, will probably already show a marked labial inclination of the upper anteriors. Frequently the upper cuspids also

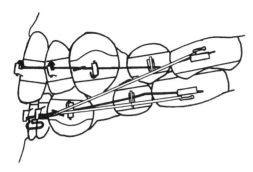

Fig. 13.5. Stage 2 space closure. A lingual root torque auxiliary can be applied to the lower incisors, near passively, to prevent excessive labial transference of the root apices. This addition will not be found necessary in the majority of treatments.

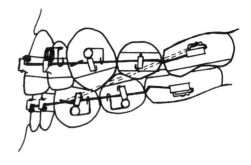

Fig. 13.6. Stage 3 root movements. This is an example and not a set pattern, as with other examples given of appliance stages. The exact method will depend on individual requirements.

show a strong mesial inclination, so that a braking action through the use of root movement auxiliaries also becomes inapplicable.

The use of Class III and lower intra-maxillary elastics for the closure of all residual space means that the lower labial segment is the sole supplier of anterior anchorage. The closure of large amounts of space could result in the lower labial segment becoming excessively lingually inclined. Before this happens, the progressive labial shift of the lower incisor apices should be arrested by the application of a lingual root torque auxiliary (*Fig. 13.5*). The auxiliary should, in this situation, be fitted near passively to prevent unwanted root movement, rather than for the purpose of apical correction.

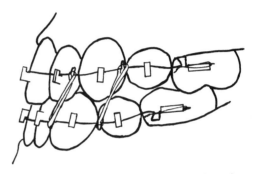

Fig. 13.7. Use of vertical elastics to assist the main archwire to seat the buccal teeth, should this be necessary at the conclusion of treatment. The same mechanical method can be used anteriorly to increase existing overbite.

Stage 3 in Treatment of Class III

An example of the mechanical arrangement of Stage 3, appropriate to a Class III treatment is shown in *Fig. 13.6*. The archwires are made of 0·020 in wire and contain the usual inter-maxillary hooks, anchor bends and toe-in. The latter bends should be of a degree adequate to compensate for the size of the buccal tube so that the forces for control of the molars against tilt or rotation are just positive.

In the treatment of Class III there will be no need to maintain overbite reduction, therefore the Stage 3 archwires will not require additional bends in the bicuspid region for the purpose of increasing the curve of Spee or, in the lower arch, to implant reverse curvature. The archwires would lie flat against any flat surface except in the area of the anchor bends. Space which has been closed in Stage 2 must be prevented from reopening during Stage 3 by any of the methods previously described.

The root movements needed will vary in accordance with the exact form of the original malocclusion and the location of subsequent extractions, if any. In most cases it will not be wise to attempt to correct fully the lingual tilt of the lower incisors or cuspids. In the case of the upper incisors, if root torque is required it will probably be for labial apical movement, see *Fig. 5.6b*. As with anterior torque archwires for palatal or lingual root movement, that for the opposite action nevertheless has the same side effect posteriorly, namely to cause arch expansion. Compensatory contraction of the auxiliary should therefore be applied.

Continuation of the use of Class III elastics may not be necessary in Stage 3, unless it has been decided that a limited amount of correction of the lower labial segment inclination can be safely carried out by lingual or distal root torque.

At the conclusion of Stage 3, it may be found, in some cases, that the incisor overbite should be increased or the buccal teeth socketed in. For the purpose of these closures, vertical elastics can be applied to 0·020 in passive archwires which carry vertical spurs over which the elastics are placed, *Fig.* 13.7. These same archwires can be used for final alignment and retention. Some orthodontists like to improve stability by using two archwires lying one above the other in each dental arch. If this is done, the archwires must be carefully coordinated in shape or inadvertant root movement can result.

It is probably true to say that those occlusions which respond successfully and permanently to closure of buccal open bite, are the same as those which would do so unaided, although the natural process might take longer. Those which do not possess the natural potential may respond to vertical elastic closure, but relapse later, wholly or partially.

In view of the whole of the preceeding text, it would seem unnecessary to give the details of the appliance mechanics which would follow the choice of teeth other than the first bicuspids for extractions. It is to be hoped that the reader will be able to work out the change in anchorage balance, as well as mechanical method, from descriptions given earlier.

Chapter 14

Local irregularities and the treatment of Class I

The opportunity will be taken in this chapter not only to describe the treatment of Class I mal-occlusion, but also to include description of some mechanical methods which can be used to deal with certain local anomalies and atypical situations, although not necessarily related to Class I.

Treatment of Class I

It is almost axiomatic that a Class I occlusion can only develop in patients whose skeletal pattern is either Class I, or mildly Class II or III. Natural compensation for minor tendency towards Skeletal II or III will be brought about by slight variations in the incisor angles, the lower incisors usually making the greater contribution. There will be no overjet, reverse overjet or overbite problems, so that the treatment of the Class I case will be mainly devoted to the elimination of the mani-festations of dental overcrowding. Extraction will probably be necessary, except in examples of very minor discrepancy, and even these would presum-ably require extraction if strict adherence to the theory of attritional occlusion is accepted.

When contemplating extraction in a Class I case, the anchorage balance struck by all possible alternative choices should be examined. Since there will be no overjet or overbite, there will be no anchorage expenditure for their correction. The usual requirement, consequently, is for the creation of space sufficient for the displaced teeth to be moved into the line of the arch with, for preference, a little to spare.

In the case of the more severe multiple tooth displacements, first bicuspid extraction would probably be justified, but, in less crowded con-ditions, the amount of space created by the same choice might prove excessive, making it difficult to obtain closure in a reasonable period of time and without over-retraction of the labial segments.

In order to close such excess residual space in the extraction sites, it would be necessary to reverse the balance of anchorage resistance by compelling bodily movement of the anteriors through the fitting of palatal or lingual root torque auxiliaries and/or cuspid uprighting springs for distal root movement. The arrangement will certainly enable the posterior teeth to be moved mesially to a far greater extent than the anteriors are retracted, but root movement of the anteriors will take place and may not always be beneficial to the result. The use of intra- and inter-maxillary space closing elastics, over a protracted period, will inevitably cause some retraction of the anteriors, in spite of the bodily control given to the latter; and this fact could be damaging to the appearance of the patient in profile. The reversal of anchorage slows the rate of movement of the anteriors relative to the posteriors, but does not prevent movement anteriorly. It is sad that, in the light of such experiences, belief in stationary anchorage must perforce be relinquished.

One way to reduce the risk of over-retracting the labial segments, or 'dishing in' of the profile, is to extract the second bicuspids rather than the first, so keeping four more teeth in the anterior anchorage. Following upon the final choice for extractions, as suited to the case under treatment, the mechanical procedures adhere to the now familiar three stage plan.

Stage 1 involves the process of general align-ment by plain or looped archwires, carrying the usual inter-maxillary hooks and mild degree anchor and toe-in bends.

Any residual extraction space is eliminated in Stage 2, using conventional Stage 2 archwire patterns. Closing elastics should include the Class II inter-maxillary rubbers, in spite of the absence of an overjet. If upper and lower intra-maxillary elastics only are used the result is liable to be more retraction of the lower labial segment than the upper, thereby creating an unwanted overjet.

Stage 3 will be devoted to the correction of the axial inclinations of those teeth which were, or have become, tilted. The Stage 3 archwires and auxiliaries, as previously described, are applicable to the Class I case.

Bimaxillary Protrusion

There are some individuals who possess a Class I relationship of the buccal teeth but whose incisors, both upper and lower, are labially inclined to an above average extent, which may spoil the general harmony of facial appearance. There is usually little malalignment of the individual teeth of such cases, space for their accommodation having been gained by the labial tilt of the incisors. Treatment will be directed mainly to the reduction of incisor prominence and better facial aesthetics, and less towards occlusal function, which may already be good. The latter, however, must not be sacrificed in the process of obtaining the former.

It should be borne in mind, when considering reduction of bimaxillary protrusions, that some are of ethnic origin. For some races a degree of bimaxillary protrusion is the natural order and over-retraction by treatment should be avoided.

In order to reduce the prominence of the incisors, space will be needed and extractions will have to be carried out for the purpose. In the absence of overjets, deep overbites or general displacement of teeth from the line of the arch, Stage 1 of treatment will be brief. The main treatment will amount to a Stage 2 space closing enterprise, wherein the labial segments are pitted against the posteriors, using the usual Z complex of intra- and inter-maxillary elastics. The anteriors are permitted to tilt freely into more acceptable angles to base, whilst the posteriors are prevented from tilting by the archwire anchor bends. The balance of anchorage resistance should be such that by the time the extraction spaces become closed the labial segments have been retracted to the desired amount.

In some instances it may be found that the above balance of tooth movement is more a theoretical than practical fact, in that the posteriors may move mesially faster than expected and, as a result, the amount of retraction of the anteriors may prove less than that which was planned. When events take this course, the failure to reduce the

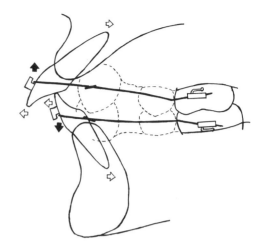

Fig. 14.1. In extremes of bimaxillary protrusion, the depression force from the main archwires to reduce overbite (black arrows) is so orientated to the long axes of the incisors that further labial tilt can occur (reaction in direction of white arrows). Space-closing elastics must overcome this tendency before becoming effective for incisor retraction. In this way the anchorage value of the labial segments can be unintentionally increased, with the possible result that the posterior segments may be moved forward to close all space, before the bimaxillary protrusion becomes adequately reduced. It may be necessary to apply limited labial root torque to upper or lower incisors, or both, in order to obtain proper intrusion and reduce strain on posterior anchorage.

bimaxillary protrusion sufficiently is often accepted as the result, for example, of an adverse lip–tongue balance. This is not necessarily so. In order to explain the true reason for this the mechanical action of the appliance should receive more detailed analysis.

In bimaxillary protrusion cases the incisors are markedly labially inclined, which means that the direction of intrusive force on the incisors derived from the anchor bends is so far from being along the long axes as to actually produce a protrusive force, which would cause the incisors to become even more labially inclined if no space closing elastics were worn. This action of the archwires effectively increases anterior anchorage, although unintentionally. The intra-maxillary elastics have to overcome this resistance before causing retraction. In addition, the Class II inter-maxillary elastics will assist in maintaining the lower labial segment position antero–posteriorly, which in turn limits the retraction of the upper. In this way the balance of resistance is shifted so that space becomes closed by the forward movement of the

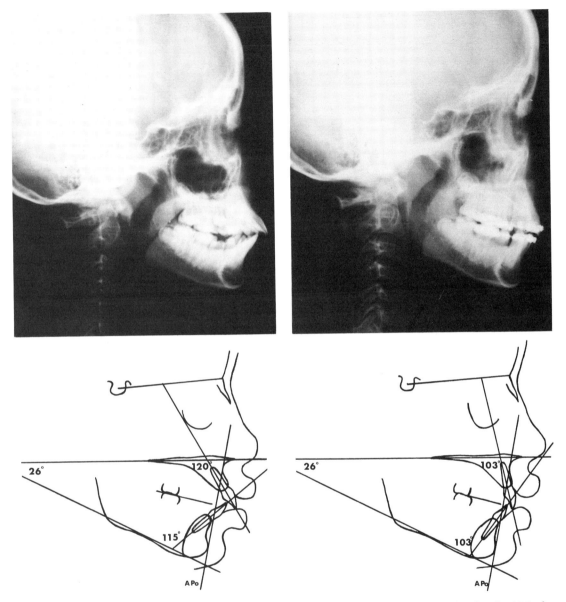

Fig. 14.2. Lateral skull of bimaxillary protrusion before treatment. Patient is of Chinese origin. Initial reaction to plain archwires was to increase the long axis angle to base of both upper and lower incisors. Labial root torque was thereafter applied to the lower incisors, whilst Class II elastics were continued to the uppers.

Fig. 14.3. The same patient as shown in *Fig.* 14.2 after two months of lower incisor labial root torque and Class II elastics. The retraction of the upper incisors has not yet caught up with that of the lowers, but the latter are now under control and the remaining reduction can be carried out without premature loss of what was a quite critical amount of lower arch anchorage, even with first bicuspid extraction.

posterior teeth with inadequate retraction of the anteriors (*Fig.* 14.1).

The above situation will only develop where incisors are labially inclined to an exceptional degree. The more upright the incisors are on base,

the nearer to their long axes the intrusive force from the archwires becomes, thus reducing the proclining effect. Indeed, when the incisors are initially near 90° to base, the same intrusive action

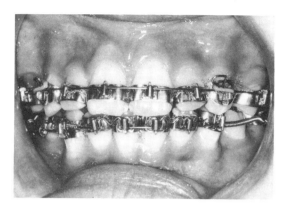

Fig. 14.4. Intra-oral view of the appliance system used for the patient shown in *Figs.* 14.2 and 14.3. The lower torque archwire is shown. The coil spring is not for the purpose of centre line correction, but is a passive length to prevent overclosure of the space for lower right 5 which was initially partially erupted. Centre line correction follows as soon as the incisors have been brought under control.

of the archwires may produce the opposite effect—retroclination.

Obviously, the inadvertent increasing of anterior anchorage in the manner described above is likely to be greater when the intrusive force on the anteriors has to be sustained over long periods in order to eliminate deep overbites. The following suggested remedy for the problem will consequently be found frequently applicable to Class II division 1 bimaxillary protrusions, as well as Class I.

If it is noticed that the labial segments are not retracting at the required rate relative to the mesial movement of the posteriors in response to the Stage 2 elastics, the lower archwire can be changed for one with M spurs anteriorly for the purpose of applying limited labial root torque to the lower incisors (*Fig.* 8.3). The lower torque archwire will upright the lower incisors without the use of an intra-maxillary elastic, so reducing the strain on lower posterior anchorage. It is probably advisable, at this stage, to use only the inter-maxillary elastics, so that the retraction of the upper incisors keeps pace with that of the lowers. It is important that the amount of labial root torque on the lower incisors be so slight as to be barely perceptible at the time the archwire is fitted, or too much movement may result (*Figs.* 14.2, 14.3 and 14.4).

The point when the intra-maxillary elastics should be reemployed is a matter for nice judgement. The object of the lower torque arch is to initiate uprighting of the lower incisors, so making

them more readily retractable, whilst an intrusive force is simultaneously operating. If this action is taken too far, closure of remaining space by elastics by conventional Stage 2 mechanics, could over-retract the labial segments, with attendant detriment to the facial profile.

Cleft Palate

The treatment of these conditions should be the object of separate study and is not within the scope of this particular book. The nature of the condition will produce the need for tooth rotation, general alignment and space closure for which the Begg appliance could be used, although other mechanical means will probably be required in addition, for such purposes as arch expansion and to correct the effects of contraction of scar tissue following surgery.

The final tooth positioning could be carried out with the Begg appliance, but no description can be given of the precise form of archwires. The designs would have to be created in each individual case from a study of the tooth movements wanted and a knowledge of the mechanical prinicples underlying the appliance action. Study of the reciprocal effects of the chosen components is, as always, worthy of greater consideration than is satisfaction with the effects of direct action alone.

Palatally Displaced Cuspids

Grossly displaced cuspids, buried in the palate, may not be recoverable by orthodontic means and will have to be either extracted or left in situ.

In a situation where the apex of the buried cuspid is in good position but the crown displaced from the line of the arch, the opportunity may exist to bring the tooth into its proper location by orthodontic means following surgical uncovering.

If the surgical procedure is properly performed, the tooth will begin to erupt, so that after a few weeks, during which healing has also taken place and the dressing removed, it should be possible to fit an attachment by direct bond to the tooth surface. It may not always be possible to gain access to that part of the tooth to which one would ideally wish to place the attachment. The initial objective will be to move the tooth towards its correct position in the dental arch, disregarding for the time being rotation and the long axis angle.

Mechanical pressure for the purpose of this

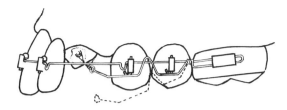

Fig. 14.5. The palatally displaced canine. The redoubling of the archwire to form a cantilever spring, adjustable as to length and direction of force application, for the repositioning of a canine crown in the line of the arch. In this instance an oval buccal tube is used to accommodate the double archwire.

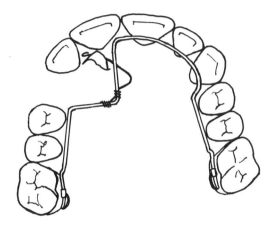

Fig. 14.6. The palatally displaced canine. The tip of the uncovered canine may be so located as to make access from the labial difficult or the apparatus liable to damage. A simple spring attached to a palatal 1 mm archwire can be useful in inaugurating the repositioning movement.

alignment can be directed from either the buccal or palatal aspect of the tooth. A useful modification of The Begg appliance for the manipulation of previously buried cuspids is shown in *Fig.* 14.5. The free arms are readily adjustable to give appropriate force directions. The reciprocal action of such adjustments on the anchor molars should be realized, particularly that which stems from a force application to bring the cuspid from the palate to the line of the arch. Reciprocally, this adjustment can cause mesio–palatal rotation of the molar. In order to avoid the undesirable effect, the amount of toe-in given to the distal of the main archwire should be slightly increased over the usual.

It is not always possible, without risk of damage to the appliance, to have access to the palatally displaced tooth from the buccal. In these circumstances a palatal archwire in 0·045 in wire carrying

auxiliary springs can be used for initial movement until access from the buccal becomes possible (*Fig.* 14.6). Final positioning is carried out by the conventional forms of archwire and auxiliaries as required.

Local Root Torque

The orthodontic repositioning of the buried cuspid often produces the need for buccal movement of the root apex. The direction of crown movement into the arch tends to displace the apex palatally. In order to correct the displacement, the form of archwire shown in *Fig.* 14.7*b* is appropriate. The

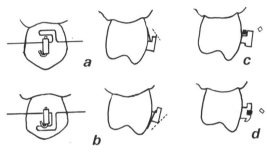

Fig. 14.7. Local root torque. *a,* Spur for palatal movement of cuspid or bicuspid root. *b,* Spur arrangement for the opposite action, i.e. buccal root movement. *c* and *d,* Alternatives for the same root movements, based on edgewise or ribbon arch mechanics, using strong milled brackets to avoid bracket distortion from the considerable forces developed by the archwires. The Begg/Chun–Hoon (*d*) is an example of a dual purpose bracket, having vertical and horizontal slots.

spur is angled so that contact is made at the tooth surface, whilst the archwire lies just proud of the bracket slot. On pinning, a torque force is set up.

When the opposite apical movement is desired, the spur is placed the other way up, to contact the tooth towards the gingival. Either arrangement is equally applicable to apical correction of bicuspids.

Treatment Mechanics
Use of Coil Springs

Coil springs are a useful accessory, mainly for two purposes: first, for the creation of space locally for the accommodation of an individual unit; and secondly for the maintenance of space between units (*Fig.* 14.4).

For the first of these purposes the coil is active. The force should be light, because of the free tilt permitted by the style of bracket, and the lumen of the coil need be little more than the gauge of the archwire. The gauge of wire used for the coil need be no more than 0·010 in. The action coil will open the space between two units, whilst closing space between the units either side. If the latter space does not exist, the action of the coil must become stultified, or the teeth imbricated.

When coils are used to maintain space they are usually applied passively, cut to the precise length required and with the helicles unopened. If support at one end is to be provided by the mesial of a buccal tube it is obviously necessary to use a coil of a size which will not be swallowed by the tube.

One advantage of the coil as a means of maintaining space is that the pattern of the archwire can be suited to a future purpose, so that, once the coil has been removed, it will not be necessary to bend a new archwire, which would be probable if space-keeping stop loops had been used. On the other hand, closed coils eventually become well loaded with putrifying food debris, so that loop stops might be reasonably regarded as the more hygienic.

Loop Stops

As an alternative to the coil, stops can be bent into the archwire to maintain arch length, or for the retention of local space. As with any loop in an archwire, unless used for root torque, there should be no contact with the tooth surface either at the time of fitting, or subsequently as a result of change of tooth position. If stop loops are placed in the anterior of an upper archwire when the upper labial segment is to be retracted, they must be bent in the plome of the archwire, or towards the occlusal. If bent in a gingival direction, contact between the stop and the tooth surface may occur as palatal tilting takes place, resulting in unintentional bodily control (see Fig. 7.2a, b and d).

Headgear

There are situations arising out of the variations with which the orthodontist has to contend where some use of extra-oral anchorage could be used with the Begg appliance to avoid over-expenditure of intra-oral anchorage or the provision of the latter by resort to multiple extraction. Possible examples have been given earlier in this text. The extra-oral force can be applied either to the anterior or posterior of the arch. In the anterior

region, application is by J hooks on the headgear arms, linked to rings on the main archwire (*Fig. 8.8*). Posterior application is by facebow fitted into supplementary tubes on the molars (*Fig. 10.5*).

It is probably better to apply the headgear to the anterior of the arch in most cases, but, if applied to the molars, it should be realized that some distal tilt of the molars is difficult to avoid when a facebow is used. If a conventional anchor bend in the main archwire is also active, the combined effect is liable to cause dramatic distal molar tilt. The use of an increased curve of Spee at least reduces the risk whilst minimizing loss of anterior overbite reduction, but does not entirely eliminate the liability.

The ease of tilt allowed by the ribbon arch style of bracket should be borne in mind when determining force application. Anchorage support should be sound with headgear forces of 250 g or less.

When the force is applied to the anterior of an arch in which all spacing has already been closed, it would be safe policy to maintain arch length by equipping the main archwire with molar stops.

The principles underlying the fitting and adjustment of extra-oral apparatus is an extensive subject in itself and considered outside the scope of this work, since it should be a matter for separate study. The information gained would be valuable wherever headgear was employed. Possible employment in conjunction with the Begg appliance would not seriously alter either mode of application or adjustment. For example, the differing force directions and consequent effects upon the upper molars, derived from alterations of the relative angle of the external arms of a Kloehn type facebow, would remain the same whether Begg or edgewise were the main appliance.

Dual Purpose Brackets

To tilt or not to tilt is a fundamental question where orthodontic appliances are concerned. Full axial control of teeth, either individually or in groups, is at times an advantage, but at others there is a call for a degree of freedom to tilt. These conflicting requirements are additional to those for directional movement.

The edgewise combination of horizontally slotted bracket and rectangular archwire represents the logical ultimate in full axial control. The vertically slotted Ribbon arch or Begg bracket is equally well suited to permit mesio–distal tilt. There are times however, during a given treatment, when whichever form of control is chosen, be it bodily or tilting, some disadvantage can be experienced. In consequence, what is sought is a system of bracket/archwire linkage, which permits the operator to exchange tilt for bodily movement at, so to speak, the turn of a switch. No such combination has yet been found suited to the restricted confines of the oral cavity.

So far most attempts to obtain the dual advantage have been based on a double slotted bracket, the one suited to Begg mechanics and the other to edgewise. It is open to argument as to whether techniques based on such brackets, have to date attained the best of both worlds or been more successful at approaching the worst of them.

The dual purpose bracket has much attraction for those whose hearts are still with edgewise mechanics. The horizontal slot and rectangular archwire can be used for final tooth positioning and bucco–lingual root correction. There are those who like to see perfection at the time the appliances are removed and to have enjoyed the precision offered them by edgewise mechanics. They like to obtain photographs of the completed result at this point, taking no risk that time might possibly show that all their precision was precisely wrong.

The fact that with the Begg appliance the final settlement of the occlusion is brought about through natural rather than artificial forces may have more to recommend it than is currently thought, so long as the appliance has been used successfully to that point.

This last observation is a most critical one. The Begg appliance and technique, in spite of apparent simplicities, is probably the most difficult of any to master to a level which produces a consistent high standard of result. Anyone reaching that level using the Begg appliance would almost certainly be able to do the same with any other method.

Although there would appear to be no long term value in final tooth positioning by edgewise mechanics, or a Stage 4 routine, there are the inevitable minority exceptions which would benefit; for example, in the treatment of a mal-occlusion in which there was gross displacement of incisor apices, the one to the buccal and the other to the lingual. Round archwires and spurs can correct the apical malplacement but, because of the severity, the appropriate auxiliary must be in place for a considerable time. The longer Stage 3 has to be continued, the more likely it becomes that small undesirable movements of anchor units may take place. The reason lies in the comparative lack of solidarity in anchorage control, over long periods, using round archwires associated with numerous active spring auxiliaries. Edgewise mechanics provide better control by what amounts to a splinting of the anchor units.

In the above and like situations, the use of rectangular wire in a Stage 4 procedure can enable the duration of the standard Stage 3 to be shortened and give the anchorage greater stability whilst the final movements are completed.

Such a procedure would represent a further modification to the standard Begg mechanics to cover certain weak areas of efficiency, and is additional to those already mentioned in the preceeding text which include:

1. The occasional use of extra-oral anchorage, either to avoid unnecessary extraction, or to help minimize extensive 'round tripping' by root apices through providing additional support during the period when torque auxiliaries are in place;

2. The use of the second permanent molar to supply vertical anchorage. It might be added that there is sometimes a discrepancy between the first permanent molar and the second at the conclusion of treatment, either laterally or vertically, and the inclusion of the second molar in the band-up may be needed for a tidy result; and

3. There are occasions when items of the mechanics of one stage should be coordinated with those of another. Although it would be desirable to avoid such amalgams in the interests of simplicity, no foul will have been committed unless principles have been offended. One should not be tied to dogma where the mechanism is concerned. It is the objectives of the three stages which should be kept separate, not necessarily the mechanics.

Chapter 15

Methods of post-treatment retention

The aim of orthodontic treatment is to so alter the occlusion that the optimum improvement is reached for the individual patient in respect of function, prevention and aesthetics. The optimum treatment result does not necessarily imply perfection, because unavoidable limitations can arise from anatomical, physiological, pathological, psychological and circumstantial issues relating to the patient. Nevertheless, whatever the standard of result, it is highly desirable that the new form of the occlusion should be stable and self-retentive and not show a tendency to revert to the original pattern.

In the long term, permanency must stem from those factors which govern the stability of the occlusion in the natural state. In the short term, however, it is seldom that the treated occlusion is given adequate support against 'relapse' by the natural factors alone. Immediately on cessation of tooth movement, the tendency to revert is marked and almost universally apparent, particularly where tooth rotation has been involved. It can readily be demonstrated that this process is no mere passive falling back to former positions, but that the teeth are actively drawn in these directions. The work of Reitan on dogs suggests that this activity comes from the fibres of the periodontal membrane and gingivae which, as a result of tooth movement, are placed on tension and disorientated. Whatever may be the cause, the activity will usually be sufficient in the first instance to overcome all natural factors which might otherwise provide stability.

In consequence, a period of artificial support, or retention, is provided for the teeth by a suitable type of passive appliance during which some rehabilitation can take place. The presence of activity, deliberate or inadvertent, within the retaining appliance will delay the process. Reitan considers that the reason for increased natural stability following this enforced rest period is the engulfing by new bone of the old periodontal fibres, thereby removing much of the tension

productive of relapse. Unfortunately, the marginal gingival fibres are not so engulfed, and show little inclination to reorientate even after several years of retention: this may be the reason for the susceptibility to relapse of tooth rotation.

It is probably unwise, with the present available knowledge and in the presence of so many variables, to offer hard and fast rules for the duration of the retention period. Fear of relapse is very real to most orthodontists and some are affected to a degree that causes them to institute retention *ad infinitum* in all treated cases without regard to individual conditions. The prospect of permanent retention is daunting to even the most cooperative patient and every effort should be made to avoid such a measure wherever possible.

In practice it is found that a small minority of treated occlusions will indeed require permanent retention. Another small minority will require no retention, whilst the majority will need a limited period, after which the factors of natural stability can be expected to be capable of sustaining the situation.

Once the initial period of tissue repair and rehabilitation is completed, the continued wearing of a retainer does not increase potential for natural stability in proportion to the time worn.

Relative Need of Individuals for Retention

In order to clarify the foregoing summary of the role of retention and be more specific in the matter of the relative need of individual patients for this measure, it would perhaps be helpful to comment further on:

1. The factors governing the stability of the occlusion in the natural state;
2. The role of various retention methods;
3. The purpose of overcorrection of tooth position;
4. The role of pericision; and
5. Modes of permanent retention.

The Natural Stability of the Occlusion

In Chapter 11 a description was given of the eruptive behaviour of the upper and lower permanent incisors. It was indicated that these teeth, before eruption, are guided towards the summit of the alveolar ridge by the peripheral cortical plates. The alveolar ridges take their shape partly from their bony foundation and partly from surface moulding from the surrounding soft tissues. The crest of the ridges can therefore be regarded as being at or near the point of equilibrium between muscular forces on either side. Consequently the permanent incisors reach eruption in positions convenient to local muscular action.

Once erupted, the crowns of the teeth become directly affected by the local musculature, which promotes a second phase of tooth positioning. After a few weeks of settling in amongst themselves, the fully erupted teeth have taken up their final positions. The resulting occlusion, whatever may be its defects, can at least be regarded as comparatively stable until such times as some event occurs, for example the loss of a unit, which upsets the former balance.

It can be reasonably inferred that what occurs in the incisor region would also apply to the buccal teeth.

Unfortunately, when alluding to the stability of tooth position, it has to be admitted that the occlusion is never entirely static. Quite apart from physical changes which may take place in the teeth themselves, or their supporting structures, there is an apparent mesial migration of the dentition which, as a continuous process, may come to affect the stability of individual units with the passage of time. The area most notably affected is the lower labial segment which, in the modern occlusion, cannot escape into an edge-to-edge relationship with the uppers because of the overbite. The continued mesial migration, in these circumstances, is one factor leading to lower incisor imbrication.

All that can be done through treatment and subsequent retention is to ensure as much stability as possible within the dentition through the use of all means available to that end.

Translating the above into terms suited to the practical orthodontist, it could be said that, ignoring displacements due to overcrowding, the general position of the teeth bucco–lingually of the whole of the lower arch and the upper buccal segments before treatment is never far from the equilibrium zone. Caution has to be exercised, in consequence, when contemplating either buccal expansion or labial movement of the lower anteriors. The lower labial segment becomes in this way a clinical guide to the antero–posterior positioning, during treatment, of the entire occlusion.

Much general alignment of the dental arches therefore has to be carried out through mesio–distal movements rather than arch expansion. Space for the mesio–distal movement will frequently have to be created by selective extractions, which also, by altering the balance within the arches, assist the ultimate stability of the result.

This does not mean that bucco–lingual tooth movement is never possible nor inadvisable. The most obvious examples of potentially stable bucco–lingual tooth movements are as follows:

(i) Teeth of the upper labial segment which have erupted onto or outside the lower lip in a position of increased overjet. An alternative position of stability usually exists for these teeth if retracted within the cover of the lower lip. The more the superior border of the lower lip overlaps the labial surface of the upper incisors, the better the prospect of stability after the retainer has been discarded. In the best circumstances, unless upper incisor rotation has been involved, the duration of retention can be relatively short.

Where no lip overlap exists, or is minimal, complete natural stability is less likely but still possible. Where the lower lip fails to act as natural retainer, it would be advisable to extend the period of artificial support. Thereafter the occlusion may yet remain stable, unless the lower lip tends to intrude under the upper incisors, or they become proclined by tongue action or digital habit.

(ii) Upper incisors may be moved from the lingual to the labial of the lower anteriors and become supported in their new position by the overbite. In the same way, crossbites in the buccal region, unless due to dental base size discrepancy, can be corrected and held by cuspal interlocking. Cuspal interdigitation however, as a factor in tooth stability, is probably often overrated.

As opposed to arch expansion, arch contraction has a better prospect of permanency, although to effect it extractions will usually have to be performed. The amount of arch contraction possible will seldom exceed 3 mm, but the reason for the stability being greater than for an equivalent amount of expansion is a matter for conjecture. An altered tongue position, or alteration in oral volumetric balance due to growth, might be in some way connected with the answer. Certainly growth is a powerful factor having much significance in the success of orthodontic treatment and the stability of the outcome.

The erupting permanent teeth take up their positions in accordance with the oral conditions which pertain at that time. Subsequent growth can alter the relative size and precise relationship of one structure to another. The direction and amount of mandibular growth is particularly significant in creating these changes.

Initial tooth position does not necessarily alter as a result of these growth changes. Indeed, the occlusal pattern, once established, remains comparatively static in most individuals. Growth however does alter potential tooth movement success by appliance, often beneficially but sometimes otherwise. For example, it can be seen in some individuals that growth has increased the width of the dental arches to an unusual extent, in others that the whole lower symphyseal region, including the lower lip, has grown forward several millimetres in relation to the cranial base or maxillary structures. This latter would help compensate for any existing overjet without affecting dental stability, unlike compensation by proclination of the lower incisors alone. The former would permit an apparent forward movement of the lower incisors to remain stable. In such ways favourable growth can assist the standard of treatment result. Where growth is unfavourable or inadequate, orthodontic measures may be made to appear less effective.

Retention Methods (*Fig.* 15.1)

The Hawley Type Removable Retainer

The Hawley type removable retainer provides a suitable passive hold following tooth movements of the simple tilting order. It supplies less reliable control over relapse following root repositioning and rotation. There is no provision for long axis control and it so happens that the cross-sectional shape of the teeth at the point where the acrylic base plate and labial archwire touch is near round, which inevitably allows some relapse of rotation.

The Begg Type Removable Retainer

The Begg type removable retainer has the same limitations as the Hawley. Its advantage is that it facilitates closure of spaces following band removal. The Begg retainer will be difficult to keep in position unless the last molars are well erupted, presenting some retentive undercut on their distal surfaces.

Removable retainers of the above patterns permit the occlusion to adjust vertically whilst offering restraint against antero–posterior or bucco–lingual relapse. The cheek teeth can erupt into full occlusal contact and the overbite can similarly adjust. If an upper retainer plate is saddled and the labial bow adjusted to hold the upper anteriors firmly against the lowers, the lower incisors will erupt, their incisal edges passing along the palatal surfaces of the uppers, until prevented from proceeding further by the degree of the inter-incisal angle, or the upper cinguli, or by the palatal soft tissues, or the tongue, or by the full expenditure of vertical growth potential of the alveolar processes.

The Kesling Type Positioner

The Kesling type positioner takes the form of a monobloc made from resilient materials. It is removable and is worn for the most part at night. Prior to construction a study is made of the original models taken before active treatment began, in order to establish the likely relapse tendencies. Then, using the final models taken at the end of the active treatment, the teeth subject to probable relapse are removed and reset in mildly overcorrected positions. The positioner is then built on the resulting mould. When the retainer is worn the teeth of both arches are held in corrected or overcorrected positions, at the same time performing the final minor adjustments with the intention of producing a more finished result.

The Barrer Spring Retainer

This design can be used to maintain alignment of the lower labial segment, or to finalize alignment of the lower incisors, following interproximal stripping to gain the required space for their

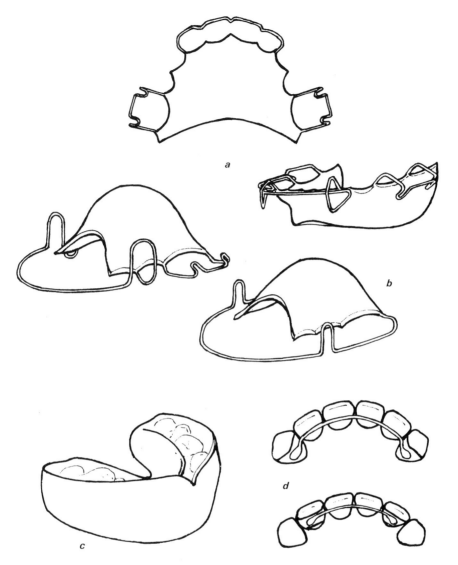

Fig. 15.1. Examples of retainer appliances. *a*, Hawley type retainers; *b*, Begg retainers; *c*, Kesling positioner; *d*, lower lingual bars.

accommodation. The retainer is made of clear acrylic so that it is unobtrusive. It can be removed and replaced easily by the patient and, in spite of its clip-on design, is stable when in position (*Fig.* 15.2).

Fixed Appliance Retention

The fixed banded type of appliance not only supplies a means of axial control of the teeth during treatment, but can also supply that same control against relapse of rotation and root correction after treatment. So long as the active period has been kept within reasonable limits, the patient may accept a few months continued wearing of the fixed apparatus in the interest of gaining the possibility of greater stability of the end result.

If this method is to be fully effective, the appliance must be completely passive, acting as a splint, and not used for tidying up operations, e.g. completion of molar rotation etc.

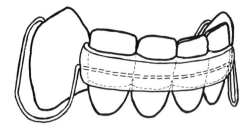

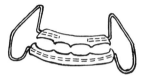

Fig. 15.2. Barrier spring retainer, made of clear acrylic so as to be unobtrusive.

The period of fixed retention should normally be followed by a further period of retention by removable appliance.

It is not always necessary for fixed retention to be supplied by the continued wearing of the entire apparatus used in the active phase. Fixed sectional retainers will often suffice, i.e. bands kept only on segments where relapse is contemplated, but removed from elsewhere, or the fitting of a lingual bar soldered to the canine or lateral incisor bands only, to support the labial segments (*see Fig.* 15.1). Direct bonding can be used to support the sectional archwires instead of bands.

Overcorrection of Tooth Position

It is advocated by some that, where practicable, a measure of overcorrection should be applied to the teeth, particularly where root movement and rotation have been involved. It is hoped in this way to compensate for initial relapse which, with no active interference, may only reach as far as the ideal position.

It is open to question whether the method produces greater stability in the long term than the provision of full correction followed by fixed passive splinting, described above. The plain advantage of overcorrection is in circumstances when the opportunity for fixed retention is prevented.

Pericision

The word pericision has been coined to describe the severing of the gingival fibres by fine knife at the root surface above the supporting bone. The operation has been performed in the hope of lessening the degree of relapse following tooth rotation and is related to Reitan's observations. It has been shown that this practice does indeed reduce initial relapse, but it is of current interest to know whether the total amount of relapse in the long term has been reduced, or whether the rate of relapse only has been slowed.

It should be remembered that not all relapse is of necessity unfavourable. Sometimes the natural effects of the local environment on the teeth, following appliance removal, are beneficial and often referred to as 'settling-in' of the occlusion. In reality this settling-in is a form of relapse which happens to favour the occlusion, but cannot otherwise be differentiated from 'relapse', which happens to be an unfavourable settling-in.

When assessing the likely relapse or settling-in probabilities of any case, the best guide will be the original models and records of the patient taken before active treatment was begun. There will always be a tendency for the original form of the occlusion to reassert itself, particularly where teeth have been rotated. The retainer must be so designed as to resist all trends towards reversion.

Finally, the natural stability factors must eventually take over. Where it is judged that these factors are not present in sufficient force, permanent retention may have to be contemplated, or some relapse accepted.

Permanent Retention

Undoubtedly there are patients whose natural retentive factors are so inadequate that an unacceptable degree of relapse can be anticipated. The only alternative is indefinite retention. Removable acrylic retainers can be used or, for additional durability, suitably designed skeleton chrome–cobalt retainers.

New bonding materials, being developed for restorative dentistry, have the prospect of providing less bulky and more convenient means of permanent support for at least some situations, and these are being added to the other alternatives.

Chapter 16

General guidance on the control of orthodontic anchorage when using the Begg appliance

When learning to use a new appliance, much early effort is directed towards reaching the requisite technical standard in constructing and fitting the various archwires and associated auxiliaries. Once accomplished, a further and even more important stage of understanding must be attained. This involves a study of the effects on anchorage of the forces set up by the archwires and other means of force production, in all their many combinations.

Observations on anchorage response to the various components of the Begg appliance have been woven into the foregoing text, together with instruction on fitting and adjustment, but the control of anchorage is of such paramount importance to the success of treatment that this chapter is devoted entirely to that topic.

There is an ever-present temptation for instructors in appliance techniques to offer well-intentioned advice through rules of thumb. Understandably, these rules relate to the typical or average situation and therefore may offer useful guidance, but in the sea of variation found within the structures forming the human individual, and the multiplicity of tooth movement problems, the average situation is inclined to occur less frequently than one might expect.

Each patient must become the object of individual thought, not just at the outset of treatment, but at every stage thereafter. Anchorage assessment must be carried out not only at the time the appliance is first fitted, but at each subsequent visit, and the apparatus adjusted accordingly. This does not call for wild improvization and invention, but for a finesse in regulating the balance of forces produced by the standard appliance components through small but important adjustment.

When using the Begg appliance events are often continuous and fast moving. The opportunity to view anchorage effects retrospectively is a privilege bestowed on the operator of slower acting appliances. The Begg appliance demands that the operator be capable of predicting accurately the forthcoming tooth movements, so that action is taken to prevent loss of anchorage before it takes place. 'Waiting to see' may be too late.

It is hoped that the following observations may be helpful when facing anchorage problems with the Begg appliance.

The Main Archwires (Stages 1 and 2)

The technical composition of Stage 1 is of deceptive simplicity. Accuracy is certainly required, but the shapes to be formed in the wire should not overtax the capability even of orthodontists of modest experience. Difficulty lies in the judgement of the force application derived through the archwire and in balancing the forces produced, so that the anchor teeth, and indeed the appliance itself, are not overstrained. Stage 1 is the most likely and also the most damaging phase of treatment in which to make any misjudgement in the above context.

The theme to be developed concerning tooth movement and anchorage control with the Begg appliance is one of determining the minimal effective forces for each separate purpose. There are those orthodontists who cannot be persuaded that, if a tooth does not move, the answer must be to use more force. Doors and windows that have jammed may respond to action based on this philosophy, but teeth move only through courtesy of bone reaction, which can differ from even resorption and deposition at the root surface with the lighter forces, to undermining resorption away from the root with the heavier. It is in connection with the latter that disadvantageous apical shift, molar rolling, root resorption and undue loss of anchorage occur, particularly with an appliance which, unlike the edgewise, does not provide full axial control. Even in the molar region the Stage 1 and 2 archwires give slender control over bodily movement by the unlikely means of a round wire in a round tube. This control can be readily overcome by the use of over-enthusiastic force application.

The object with Stage 1 and 2 archwires, should be to maintain a steady rate of improvement using minimal effective forces. There will be a maximum safe speed of tooth movement which, judged on a visit-to-visit basis, may appear to some to be slow. A temptation may be to speed matters up by increasing the inter-maxillary forces, theoretically balanced by a compensatory increase in the anchorage control bends. If this type of action is taken too far, the result may well be to slow down treatment progress by causing inadvertent tooth movements of the disadvantageous forms mentioned in the preceding paragraph. Time will have to be expended on recovery from error instead of progress, which is perhaps the commonest way of unnecessarily protracting the period of active treatment.

Initial Stage 1 Archwire

The initial Stage 1 archwire may well have as its prime purpose the general alignment of the teeth, both in the horizontal and vertical dimensions. Loops incorporated for this purpose should be kept to a minimum and used lightly active. Bracket binding can occur when loops are used in the buccal region, or when straightening grossly malaligned incisors. It may be good policy to allow the worst of the malalignment to correct before commencing Class II elastics. For example, if there is bracket binding in the upper incisor region the upper labial segment will offer greater resistance to retraction and will consequently make greater demand on lower posterior anchorage than usual, thereby expending anchorage to poor effect.

The above pre-Stage 1 procedure should be of relatively short duration. The leverage supplied to the molar teeth through modestly active anchor bends should be sufficient to maintain arch length and prevent mesial migration of the molars.

If and when doubt exists, molar stops can be incorporated.

Multi-looped and Multi-strand Archwires

Multi-looped archwires, because of their flexibility, tend to be less effective in anchorage control than plain archwires. Consequently they should be discarded as soon as their purpose has been attained. The same can be said, even more emphatically, concerning multi-strand archwires. If used at all, they should never be employed in association with inter- or intra-maxillary elastics and never for more than a week or two, for the eventual purpose of more conveniently seating a looped arch.

Inter-maxillary Hooks

The inter-maxillary hooks, both anterior and posterior, must be readily accessible to the patient, who should experience no difficulty, after initial instruction, in applying the rubbers. It is immaterial whether the Z hook or the ring type is used in Stage 1. If the Z pattern is employed, it must be angled to the plane of the archwire so that the distal arm of the hook cannot enter the slot of the canine bracket, thus inadvertently causing bodily control over that tooth and thereby adversely affecting the anchorage balance. If the ring type hook is preferred, arch form may be more difficult to obtain than with the Z loop. When using the ring hook the wire must be worked so that there is no tendency for the ring to spring open and so alter the molar width. It must also be seen that the archwire immediately to the mesial and distal of the ring continues in an even curve and does not remain relatively straight in these areas.

Anchor Bend

The purpose of the anchor bends is to supply bodily control over the molars whilst reciprocally supplying a depressive force to the anteriors. The amount of force given is fairly critical for the best effects and the force will vary with both the degree of the bend and also the antero—posterior positioning of the bend. The anchor bends are initially placed 5—6 mm in front of the mesial of the buccal tubes on each side of the upper and lower archwires. The amount of bend is best assessed·by measuring the force developed when the archwire is brought to the slots of the anterior brackets. The bends are increased until the force reaches the region of 50 g.

Toe-in Bends

Toe-in bends are not usually required during Stage 1, because, even when lightly active, the anchor bends tend to roll slightly in the buccal tubes, thus providing anti-rotational toe-in automatically. It follows that if an operator should find that he needs to toe the distal ends of the archwire out, in order to prevent molar rotation, his anchor bends are too severe and should be reduced. When this is done there will be no further need for the toe-out bends, since they were merely in compensation for an error.

Offset Bends

Offset bends in the horizontal plane can usually be avoided. There is no call for the molar offset in Stages 1 or 2, but the bicuspid offset can be of value in certain circumstances. It will be found that, when the second bicuspid has been banded, in some dental arches the archwire bears on the bicuspid bracket whilst standing to the buccal of the cuspid bracket. Once engaged in the cuspid bracket, forces are set up that would cause canine expansion and also the movement of the bicuspid lingually or palatally. A bicuspid offset bend, placed well to the mesial of the bicuspid bracket in the extraction site, will allow the archwire to be seated passively in the cuspid brackets and against the surface of the bicuspid bracket. The bends should not be greater than strictly required for this purpose.

In order to avoid molar width contraction or roll during Stage 1, the archwires are kept expanded in the molar region by 1 cm in the lower arch and by half that amount in the upper. This expansion is obtained by slightly decreasing the anterior archwire curvature. It might be thought that cuspid expansion would result, but it must be realized that the object of arch expansion is not to create an arch width increase, but to prevent the opposite. When therefore the archwires have been adjusted in the above manner and placed in the buccal tubes, it should be found that the cuspid brackets can be passively engaged. If any compression of the archwires is needed to engage the cuspid brackets, the adjustment to create expansion

in the molar region will have been incorrectly carried out. Incidentally, it is better to err on the side of over- rather than under-expansion in the molar region, and gradually to adjust to requirements through close observation of results.

Stage 2

During the second stage of treatment the amount of anchor bend and expansion is often reduced, but positive pressure must be maintained to prevent loss of overbite reduction. There are those who prefer 0·018 in archwires for this purpose, but there would appear to be little advantage over 0·016 in.

Inter- and Intra-Maxillary Elastics

As with the force applications through the archwires, the amount of force transmitted by the inter- or intra-maxillary elastics, should be kept as light as is consistent with steady progress. A force from the elastics of 60–70 g is usually advocated, although it will often be found that 50 g or even less is sufficient. Heavier forces, far from increasing the rate of tooth movement, tend to slow the process down.

If teeth fail to respond, mechanical obstruction or malfunction of the appliance should first be considered, e.g. archwire binding, contact between the distal ends of the archwire and the second molars, cuspal interference etc. Increasing pressure should be the last thing to be considered, and certainly it should seldom exceed the 70 g level. If tooth movement fails at this point, it is probable that a mechanical fault has not yet been detected, or patient cooperation has lapsed, or an anatomical obstruction has been reached.

There was a time when the necessary light forces were obtained by the use of rubber bands manufactured for office stationery purposes. This type of rubber readily absorbs moisture in the mouth and consequently swells. Over a period of five day' continuous wear an initial force of 60 g would fall considerably as the ring enlarges. There were however, some shortcomings inherent in this type of elastic:

1. When first placed in the mouth, they had a strong and not particularly pleasant taste;
2. Their colour was light to dark brown, which was detrimental to appearance when worn in an area of the mouth which could be readily seen during social encounter;

3. They were comparatively thick in cross-section and became thicker with use, requiring inter-maxillary hooks to be of the Z pattern in preference to the alternative of oversized rings; and

4. Although initial pressure might be light and, with the process of swelling even lighter, the force delivered by this type of elastic tended to build up rapidly as the patient opened his mouth.

Thin latex rubbers have been introduced which aim to overcome the above disadvantages. These also swell in the mouth, but to a lesser degree. An initial force of 60 g does not therefore reduce as much over a period of wear, as with the stationery type of rubber bands.

The rise and fall of pressure as the patient opens and closes the mouth is less with the latex variety. An average elastic ring of 8 mm diameter, made for stationery purposes, stretched to give a force of 50 g will, on being stretched a further centimetre, exert a force of 140 g. A similar dimension latex band stretched to give the same initial force of 50 g can be deflected 3 cm before the force rises to 140 g. The patient is consequently far less consciously aware of the presence of this type of elastic which, together with the other factors mentioned, makes for greater potential cooperation.

The use of the proper force values and force balance will greatly assist the quality of tooth movement obtained during Stage 1. The following is a summary of some of the desirable effects of the lighter forces as against the detrimental consequences of those in excess of the ideal:

(i) Light forces will cause movement at an acceptable rate among teeth which are permitted to tilt freely whilst being insufficient to overcome the resistance offered by anchor teeth compelled to move bodily. If the forces are raised too much, the posterior mechanical bodily control through round archwire and buccal tube will be strained beyond its somewhat tenuous limits, resulting in undue consumption of anchorage, molar tilt, rolling and rotation.

(ii) In the case of overjet reduction, the use of light inter-maxillary forces will not only have the above desirable consequences in the molar region, but also equally valuable ones in the upper labial segment. When balanced with the intrusive force

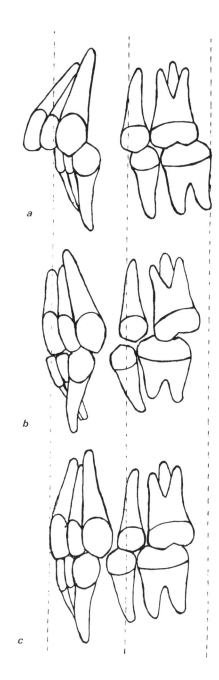

Fig. 16.1. *a* Hypothetical situation following first premolar extraction, but prior to appliance therapy. *b* Possible response of occlusion (in *a*) to Stage 1 of treatment, during which excess force has been applied through Class II inter-maxillary elastics and anchor bends, coupled with some wrong positioning of the latter. *c* Response of occlusion (in *a*) to light forces during Stage 1, avoiding the apical disorientation, root resorption and anchorage loss depicted in (*b*).

supplied by the main archwire, the upper anteriors will retract with little or no labial displacement of their apices. Too much inter-maxillary force causes more labial apical movement relative to crown retraction, resulting in unnecessary upper incisor retroclination with possible accompanying root resorption if they should become pressed against the labial cortical plate.

(iii) The result of the use of proper inter-maxillary elastic force should be seen to be bodily forward movement of the anchor molars, which in turn depends on the correct force application from the anchor bends. Increasing the degree of anchor bends to compensate for over-enthusiastic inter-maxillary elastic forces, will cause a distal tilt of the molars to become established. In the longer term, the combination of these excessive forces may bring about molar tilt, rotation and extrusion and probably root resorption.

(iv) Excessive force application from the anchor bends may cause unacceptable mobility, not only of the molars but also, through reciprocal action, the incisors. This fault is most frequently introduced in patients whose overbites prove reluctant to reduce. The operator is tempted to the conclusion that the required reduction can only be brought about by increasing the depression force, thus not only creating tooth mobility but also probably reducing the prospects of further improvement of overbite (*Fig.* 16.1).

Anchorage Factors in Stage 3

Stage 3 anchorage concerns the action and counter-action of the torquing and uprighting auxiliaries used to correct root positions. The main arch-wires act in the less active role of maintaining arch from and crown position acquired in Stage 1 and 2.

The forces derived from the root movement auxiliaries are inevitably great, by comparison with forces employed in the early stages of treatment, but this is no reason for overtaxing the anchorage. One must look once more for the minimum force for the maximum movement. One must be aware that, beyond a certain point, heavier forces may produce no increased rate of movement in desirable places, but may well produce movement where it is not required. It must be recalled that if an

auxiliary is fitted to create root movement in one direction, the crown of that tooth will move in the opposite direction.

Upper Torquing Auxiliaries

When an upper torquing auxiliary is employed for palatal root movement of the incisors, there will not only be a drag on anchorage towards the anterior, but also a tendency to expand the arch in the posterior region. The greater the force delivered by the auxiliary, the greater the risk of these detrimental effects.

In order to avoid arch expansion in the upper molar region, the torque auxiliary is contracted and also, in some people's hands, the main arch-wire needs to be also contracted to variable degrees.

Such compensatory action can be minimized by keeping down the torque force. In order to do this and to standardize the amount of force in each case, the torque spurs are applied to the incisors at an angle of no more than 40° to the long axis of their roots.

It is as well to contract all anterior torque arches, whether upper or lower and regardless of their main purpose, if molar expansion is to be avoided.

Root-Paralleling Springs

The action of root-paralleling springs also makes demand on anchorage. As with torque spurs, when the root apex is moved in one direction, the crown of that tooth will be moved in the other.

The force delivered by a paralleling spring can vary because of the size or number of the hellicles, metallurgical qualities of the wire and the length and deflection of the free arm. It will help considerably in their control, and in the predictability of the outcome of their use, if each spring is made to an identical size and shape. If their construction is inconsistent, action and reaction will be equally inconsistent, which will reduce the value of experience.

After standardizing the form of the spring, the next standardization relates to the deflection of the free arm. An 0·014 in spring is usually active to the desired amount when the free arm makes an angle with the main archwire of 45°. Obviously such a rule of thumb can only provide general guidance and the individual operator will have to adjust in accordance with personal experience.

Direction of Movement

In many instances, the required root movements will happen to be in opposite directions and may largely counteract one another, thus offsetting the possibility of creating disadvantageous shift of the dental arch; but this is by no means always so. For example, first molar extraction cases often result in the cuspid and bicuspids of each arch being distally inclined at the conclusion of Stage 2. The apices of all these teeth require distal movement of their roots in Stage 3, which will threaten to move the arches mesially to a greater extent than would be the case where there was some cancellation of the root movement forces. One means of reducing the risk would be to place a reverse torque auxiliary on the lower anteriors, in the first instance almost passively in order to give bodily control of these teeth against shift of the lower arch anteriorly from either Class II elastics or the combined effect of the uprighting auxiliaries.

One must be constantly aware that both anterior torque arches and uprighting auxiliaries can act in the capacity of brakes against unwanted movement of the dental arches. The fitting of the lower torque arch, mentioned above, is one example. In the same sense, upper or lower lingual torque arches can be placed to prevent undue retraction or retroclination of the labial segments. This is the principle under-lying the so-called 'reversal of anchorage'.

The placement of uprighting springs for distal movement of the cuspid roots will also assist the stabilization of the labial segment as a whole against forces of retraction.

In the case of the typical four bicuspid extraction situation in Stage 3, the mesial movement of the second bicuspid apices may be complete before the required distal movement of the canine apices has been accomplished, and some might be tempted to remove the bicuspid springs. It would, however, be good policy to leave them in situ to act in a braking capacity against mesial arch movement in reaction to the canine springs. Similarly it would be advisable, when continuing distal movement of the canine apex on one side of the arch, not to remove the spring used for the

same purpose on the other, as otherwise a shift of centre line may occur.

Conclusion

It is still good basic policy to keep the stages of treatment separate, but, with increasing experience and understanding of anchorage problems with the Begg appliance, there may be occasions when elements of one Stage can be successfully amalgamated with another at the discretion of the operator.

The art of handling orthodontic anchorage is the capacity to judge total tooth movement response from the forces promoted at any one time and the resistance given by the passively held units so that, by suitable appliance adjustment, the balance of movement favours treatment objectives.

The Begg appliance differs in many respects from the edgewise, the differences largely arising from the opposing forms of bracket-to-archwire linkage. The horizontal bracket slot of the edgewise appliance can provide full axial control: the vertical slot of the Begg bracket allows tilting. If the forces employed with edgewise mechanics become excessive, anchorage may be lost; but at least the axial control of the bracket slot will prevent sudden and detrimental tilting. The rate of anchorage loss will be relatively slow, giving the operator the opportunity to intervene before the situation becomes out of hand.

The bodily control balance of anchorage in edgewise techniques consume intra-oral anchorage rather readily, as a result of which extra-oral support from headgear usually has to be called upon. Such a form of anchorage is virtually inexhaustible. These factors make edgewise mechanics safer than Begg in the hands of those whose appreciation of intra-oral anchorage has not yet been sufficiently developed.

For those who can reach the necessary standards, the Begg appliance offers an economy in intra-oral anchorage expenditure in that bodily control can be provided to the anchor teeth, whether posterior or anterior, whilst other teeth are allowed to tilt. Light forces in these circumstances, cause rapid crown movement among the teeth free to tilt, whilst the same forces applied to the bodily-controlled teeth cause only small amounts of movement.

Once the third stage of treatment is reached, root repositioning is carried out whilst both upper and lower dental arches are bound together in mutual support, thereby providing anchorage which, in most instances, will be enough for the purpose without undue shift of the arches labially. The fact that root movements are often self-cancelling assists anchorage conservation.

By reason of its economic use of intra-oral anchorage, the Begg appliance rarely needs extra-oral support, unless mistakes and misjudgements have taken place. If headgear should become necessary, high or straight pull can be applied either to the front or, if suitable precaution is taken, the posterior of the arch.

The inadvertent or unavoidable full expenditure of intra-oral anchorage should not automatically invoke thoughts of the Stone Age, and of additional extraction as the only means of continuing the case to completion.

The very mechanical composition of the Begg appliance invites the use of light forces if breakdown is to be avoided, quite apart from the improved quality of tooth movement which the lighter forces produce.

The Begg appliance is both comprehensive and versatile, but it is only an instrument which, like a musical one, can be played to good effect only by those with the talent, training and perseverence to do so. Discord and disharmony will haunt those who do not possess these characteristics. It is the operator, not the appliance, who produces the results, acceptable or otherwise, directly in accordance with his ability.

Suggested reading

Adler T. (1969) Increasing posterior force vectors in Begg treatment procedures. *Begg J. Orthod.* **5**, 7–16.

Angle E. H. (1907) *Treatment of Malocclusion of the Teeth.* (7th ed.) Philadelphia, The S. S. White Manufacturing Co.

Ballard C. F. (1966–7) The morphological bases of prognosis determination and practical treatment planning. *Trans. Br. Soc. Study Orthod.* pp. 95–105.

Barrer H. G. (1967) Elastic thread with the Begg Technique. *J. Pract. Orthod.* **1**, 122–123.

Barrer H. G. (1969) Nonextraction treatment with the Begg Technique. *Am. J. Orthod.* **56**, 365–378.

Barrer H. G. (1975) Protecting the integrity of mandibular incisor position. *J. Clin. Orthod.* **9**, 486–494.

Begg P. R. (1938) Progress report of observations on attrition of the teeth in its relation to pyorrhea and tooth decay. *Aust. J. Dent.* **42**, 315–320.

Begg P. R. (1954) Stone Age man's dentition. *Am. J. Orthod.* **40**, 298–312, 373–383, 462–475, 517–531.

Begg P. R. (1956) Differential force in orthodontic treatment. *Am. J. Orthod.* **42**, 481–510.

Begg P. R. (1961) Light archwire technique. *Am. J. Orthod.* **47**, 33–48.

Begg P. R. (1962) Questions and answers. *Begg J. Orthod.* **1**, 55–62.

Begg P. R. (1963) Questions and answers. *Begg J. Orthod.* **2**, 31–35.

Begg P. R. (1968) The origin and progress of the light wire differential force technique. *Begg J. Orthod.* **4**, 9–34.

Begg P. R. and Kesling P. C. (1977) *Begg Orthodontic Theory and Technique.* (3rd ed.) Philadelphia, W. B. Saunders & Co.

Bjork A. (1967) The face in profile. *Sven. Tandläk. Tidskr.* **40**, Suppl. 5B.

Brandt S. (1962) Experiences with the Begg Technique. *Angle Orthod.* **32**, 150–166.

Broadbent B. H. (1931) A new X-ray technique and its application to orthodontists. *Angle Orthod.* **1**, 45–66.

Brodie A. G. (1944) Does scientific investigation support the extraction of teeth? *Am. J. Orthod. Oral Surg.* **30**, 445–460.

Cadman G. R. (1975) A vade mecum for the Begg Technique: Technical principles and treatment procedures. *Am. J. Orthod.* **67**, 477–512, 601–624.

Cadman G. R. (1975) Non-extraction treatment with the Begg Technique. *Am. J. Orthod.* **68**, 481–498.

Campe G., Marcus M. I. and Margolis H. I. (1967) Comparative analysis on reduction of overbite using removable appliance, Begg treatment and Tweed treatment. *Am. J. Orthod.* **53**, 150–151. Abstract.

Downs W. B. (1948) Variations in facial relationships; their significance in treatment and prognosis. *Am. J. Orthod.* **34**, 812–840.

Downs W. B. (1956) Analysis of dento-facial profile. *Angle Orthod.* **26**, 191–212.

Fletcher G. G. T. (1963) A cephalometric appraisal of the development of malocclusion, Part 1. *Trans. Br. Soc. Stud. Orthod.* 124–130.

Fletcher G. G. T. (1975) The retroclined upper incisor. *Br. J. Orthod.* **2**, 207–216.

Grieve G. W. (1944) Anatomical and clinical problems involved where extraction is indicated in orthodontic treatment. *Am. J. Orthod. Oral Surg.* **30**, 437–443.

Gould I. E. (1957) Mechanical principles in extra-oral anchorage. *Am. J. Orthod.* **43**, 319–333.

Hodgson D. W. (1968) A Class III treatment with the Begg Appliance. *J. Prac. Orthod.* **2**, 304–305.

Holdaway R. A. (1956) Changes in relationship of points A and B during orthodontic treatment. *Am. J. Orthod.* **42**, 176–193.

Howes A. E. (1947) Case analysis and treatment planning based upon the relationship of tooth material to its supporting bone. *Am. J. Orthod. Oral Surg.* **33**, 499–533.

Huckaba G. W. (1952) The physiological basis of relapse. *Am. J. Orthod.* **38**, 335–349.

Kesling H. D. (1945) The philosophy of the tooth positioning appliance. *Am. J. Orthod. Oral Surg.* **31**, 297–304.

Kesling H. D. (1956) The diagnostic set-up with consideration for the third dimension. *Am. J. Orthod.* **42**, 740–748.

Kesling P. C. (1962) A general consideration of the first stage of Begg treatment. *Begg J. Orthod.* **1**, 47–53.

Kesling P. C. (1963) Causes of loss of anchorage in first and second stages. *Begg J. Orthod.* **2**, 23–30.

Kloehn S. J. (1953) Orthodontics—Forces or persuasion. *Angle Orthod.* **23**, 56–65.

Levin R. I. (1977) Treatment results with the Begg Technique. *Am. J. Orthod.* **72**, 239–260.

Margolis H. I. (1943) The axial inclination of mandibular incisors. *Am. J. Orthod. Oral Surg.* **29**, 571–594.

Marx R. (1976) High pull Begg. *Br. J. Orthod.* **3**, 169–173.

McDowell C. S. (1967) The hidden force. *Angle Orthod.* **37**, 109–131.

Mulie R. M. and Ten Hoeve A. (1976) The effect of antero–posterior incisor positioning on the palatal cortex as studied with laminagraphy. *J. Clin. Orthod.* **10**, 804–822.

Mulie R. M. and Ten Hoeve A. (1976) The limitations of tooth movement within the symphysis, studied with laminagraphy and standardized occlusal films. *J. Clin. Orthod.* **10**, 882–899.

Ten Hoeve A., Mulie R. M. and Brandt S. (1977) Technique modifications to achieve intrusion of the maxillary anterior segment. *J. Clin. Orthod.* **11**, 174–198.

Nance H. N. (1947) The limitations of orthodontic treatment. *Am. J. Orthod. Oral Surg.* **33**, 177–223, 253–301.

Oppenheim A. (1944) A possibility of physiological ortho-dontic movement. *Am. J. Orthod. Oral Surg.* **30**, 277–328, 344–368.

Ricketts R. M. (1960) A foundation for cephalometric communication. *Am. J. Orthod.* **46**, 330–357.

Reitan K. (1967) Clinical and histologic observations on tooth movement during and after orthodontic treat-ment. *Am. J. Orthod.* **53**, 721–745.

Rodesano A. J. (1974) Treatment of Class III malocclusion with the Begg light wire technique. *Am. J. Orthod.* **65**, 237–245.

Sims M. R. (1962) The Begg philosophy and treatment technique. *Begg J. Orthod.* **1**, 23–36.

Sims M. R. (1971) Anchorage variation with the light wire technique. *Am. J. Orthod.* **59**, 456–469.

Smith R. and Storey E. (1952) The importance of force in orthodontics. *Aust. J. Dent.* **56**, 291–304.

Storey E. and Smith R. (1952) Force in orthodontics and its relation to tooth movement. *Aust. J. Dent.* **56**, 11–18.

Smyth K. C. (1934) Some notes on the dentitions of Anglo-Saxon skulls from Bidford-on-Avon, with special reference to malocclusion. *Dent. Rec.* **54**(1), 1.

Steiner C. (1953) Cephalometrics for you and me. *Am. J. Orthod.* **39**, 729–755.

Swain B. F. (1969) In: Graber T. M. (ed.), *Current Ortho-dontic Concepts and Technique* (1st ed.), Vol. 2. Philadelphia, Saunders. pp. 585–816.

Swain B. F. and Ackerman J. L. (1969) An evaluation of the Begg technique. *Am. J. Orthod.* **55**, 668–687.

Tweed C. H. (1946) The Frankfort–Mandibular plane angle in orthodontic diagnosis, classification, treatment planning and prognosis. *Am. J. Orthod. Oral Surg.* **32**, 175–221.

Williams R. (1968) The cant of the occlusal plane and mandibular plane with and without pure Begg treat-ment. *J. Pract. Orthod.* **2**, 496–505.

Williams R. (1969) The diagnostic line. *Am. J. Orthod.* **55**, 458–476.

Williams R. (1970) Begg treatment of high angle cases. *Am. J. Orthod.* **57**, 573–589.

Direct Bonding

The bonding of brackets direct to the tooth surfaces, avoiding the use of bands, has advanced in popularity in harmony with improvements in bonding materials, techniques for application and increased reliability.

Amongst the advantages to be gained by the method is one of considerable reduction in the chairside time required to initially equip a patient with the full apparatus.

The time estimates given in the foregoing account, relating to the fitting of bands, would be changed by the use of direct bonding, but not the principles governing bracket placement.

Description has been given in relation to the use of bands, because that method has not been completely superseded and can still be preferred particularly where lingual attachments are needed.

Every precaution should be taken to avoid breakdown of either bands or bonds and consequent loss of control over the tooth or teeth which, with luck, may only be partial in the case of the loss of a cement lining of a band but total in the case of the failure of a direct bond.

Index

Terms used in this index refer to the Begg Appliance in general
and to Class II division 1 occlusions except where indicated.